From

ALZHEIMER'S

With Love

From ALZHEIMER'S With Love

A Remarkable Journey of Healing through the Grace of Jesus

Marc Swift

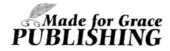

Made for Grace
PUBLISHING

Made for Success Publishing
P.O. Box 1775
Issaquah, WA 98027

From Alzheimer's With Love

Designed by Dee Dee Heathman
Postcard Cover Concept by Marc Swift

Scripture quotations are taken from *The Living Bible*, © 1971 by Tyndale House Foundation. Used by permission of Tyndale House Publishers, Inc., Carol Stream, Illinois 60188, and the *New King James Version* © 1982 by Thomas Nelson. Used by permission. All rights reserved.

Library of Congress Cataloging-in-Publication data

Swift, Marc
    From Alzheimer's With Love: A Remarkable Journey of Healing
    Through the Grace of Jesus / Marc Swift
    p. cm.
    ISBN-13: 978-1-61339-878-4 (pbk.)
    LCCN: 2016914179
    PCIP: LCC BV4910.9 .S95 2017 | DDC 242.4--dc23

LCSH: Swift, Marc--Family. | Healing--Religious aspects--Christianity. | Spiritual healing. | Alzheimer's disease--Patients--Family relationships. | Alzheimer's disease--Patients--Care. | Fathers and sons.

To contact the publisher please email service@MadeforSuccess.net or call +1 425 657 0300.

Made for Grace in an imprint of Made for Success Publishing.
Printed in the United States of America

Praise for *From Alzheimer's With Love*

———————— ✿ ————————

This is a really, really good book! Having known Marc for a number of years now, and having listened to many of his stories, I have witnessed his growth in faith and faithfulness. The story of his Dad being freed through deliverance prayer will lead us to consider how the demonic affects the body, soul, and spirit of the Alzheimer's patient. There certainly is a place for bold prayer. For many, these are uncharted waters, but Marc presents this information in a way that encourages us to give it a try.

—Pastor Steve Horrell,
The Healing Ministry at All Saints Church

Marc Swift's latest book, *From Alzheimer's With Love*, takes the reader on an emotionally raw and at times humorous heartfelt spiritual journey with his father. I would highly recommend this book to anyone who is now dealing with this devastating disease and needs a refreshing spiritual perspective. As Marc seeks innovative pathways of healing for his father, he introduces a wonderful approach he calls a "Guided Interactive Visualization Exercise" as a way to reach the life in the heart and the body when the mind is not there.

—Donna Oland, RN

From Alzheimer's With Love presents a very positive outlook on things. It is an excellent faith-based approach to Alzheimer's. The Christian outlook will be greatly beneficial. I highly recommend this excellent book.

—**Robert A. Cambridge,**
M.D., Neurologist

The author's "Guided Interactive Visualization Exercise" approach engagingly employs the powerful use of story to tap into one's richest life experiences to bring about healing and restoration.
—**The Rev. Cameron Nations+ Priest Associate,**
All Saints Episcopal Church

I highly recommend Swift's well-done book, *From Alzheimer's With Love*. My dear mum has it [Alzheimer's], this book helped me see deeper into the issues that rest on family members and on the patient. I read a prayer that an Alzheimer's patient wrote that really spoke to me, as Swift's book did, "Lord I don't know where I am, I don't know who I am, I don't know what I am, but please, please Love me." I think that summarizes this dreadful disease. Stand on the gift of hope.
—**The Rev. Nigel W.D. Mumford+ Priest Associate for Prayer**
Ministry, Galilee Church
Founder: The Welcome Home Initiative
© Founder and president:
By His Wounds, Inc.© Healing Ministry

An amazingly well-written story of a potentially sad situation that brought me to tears and then to triumph. Never a dull moment as I read this book. I am now inspired to embrace the relationship that I have with my family—young and old—because of the reality check that I experienced. I, too, have a wonderfully seasoned father. I am determined to enjoy every moment of life that I can with him. Parents bring so much love to our lives. This book is a reminder for me: like seeing myself in the mirror. *From Alzheimer's With Love* has great value. It is a must read.

—**Kerry Austin,**
Author and Professional Speaker

TO DAD

CONTENTS

THE BLESSING OF THE FATHER

"Escape From Alzheimer's" is a title I considered for this book. I chose not to use it because I considered it misleading, like 'back to normal after a bout of the flu.'

But even though it was a title that needed too much explaining, my dad did escape the prison of his own isolation.

I got the thought from "Escape From Alcatraz," the Clint Eastwood movie. Alcatraz was a prison island hopelessly cut off from the world, from people, from everyday life.

To think that once you were there, you would *never*, never be able to enjoy loving relationships or fun times, no longer have the freedom to enjoy the sunshine and nature, or your house, and never be with a family in your life again. Basically an image of hell, separation from Love, from God — the reason Jesus came, to reunite us with eternal Love.

My dad is becoming isolated. He is disconnecting with his memory and losing his identity as a child of God and as a beloved son of the Father.

Living with my mom, he shows few signs of having faith and though he can be pleasant and nice, he is becoming more defiant and contrary.

The deterioration and lack of communication caused by the Alzheimer's disease, already in its third year, makes my mom feel that my dad is drifting further away from her and becoming too hard to reach.

In the action adventure movie, "Escape From Alcatraz," the man escapes and lives.

In my action adventure version, "Escape From Alzheimer's," my father escapes and lives.

My dad becomes a responsive man, at peace with himself, interacting with me, smiling and laughing, answering 'yes' or 'no' to my questions, even throwing a football back and forth with me. He reconnects with me, with his beloved wife, with himself and with God.

As the last page of his life is turned, Bob Swift is restored to dignity and self-worth. He ends his life with an angel coming to get him, as we shall see. What a blessing that is!

Well, it is time to begin this story of the amazing months that led up to my father finishing his life with courage and honor. And connecting with us from Alzheimer's, with love.

PRAY FOR DAD

My father used to love scripture.

After I became a 'born-again' Catholic in 1978, my mother and father followed suit. My father grew so passionate about memorizing Scripture that he used large index cards and wrote down in his small handwriting numerous scriptures which he then set to memory.

Now my father cannot remember much at all. My father has the disease called Alzheimer's.

Lately, when I call my parents, my mother shares with me her pain of Dad talking about "the equipment." She doesn't understand what he's talking about. He's always saying: "Where is the equipment?" or "I need to do something with the equipment," or "It all depends on the equipment."

"Will you please pray for Dad, Marc?" my mom asks me in frustration. "I know you're really good about praying for healing. Pray for his brain to work again."

Six months ago I decided I could be more flexible with my schedule and actually go to Florida, stay a few days, and give my mom a break. Since then, I've been flying to Orlando every seven weeks to give my mom some relief, as she is getting tired of taking care of my father.

Thanksgiving is coming. The leaves are falling from the giant pecan trees in my yard. The air is crisp and colder than usual at this time of year. Already there is a huge pile around the Cottonwood tree in the back corner of the yard, which I call the Grandfather Tree.

I have the house to myself now and I have been singing praises while playing my guitar. I have been rejoicing because the book I spent almost three years working on is done. My book about my son, Josh, which is now published on Amazon. I began writing it shortly after Josh died peacefully in his sleep, two years and eight months ago. It is the story of our healing as a father and a son, thanks to the unconditional love of God, and the huge life-changing miracle we experienced in our relationship.

With Josh no longer living in the house by my side, writing has become the main purpose and joy of my life, while improving cars and detailing them to look like new again is my profession. Jesus healed me from a deadly brain tumor in 1977, and ever since I have been involved with healing and been passionate about the Holy Spirit.

When I am not writing, I am working on detailing cars. My helper, Shon, does the interiors and I do the exteriors. This will be the 25th year since I have set up shop in the huge garage of my home in an out of the way cul-de-sac, centrally located in Tulsa, Oklahoma.

In days of old, my two strong sons, Joshua and Michael helped me detail cars. "Idle hands are the devil's workshop," I had been told by an older Christian friend so from a young age I taught them both the art of detailing in the spirit of excellence, and they helped me after school.

Fathering them each day, as we worked together and talked, was the highlight of my life. I gave them scriptures to memorize from the Psalms, and the Gospels and the letters of Paul, Peter, John, and James. I asked them to memorize daily amounts and each verse they learned, I learned with them.

Now Shon is helping me and drawing out of me all the communication and mentoring skills that make me thrive. I have been helping him overcome a hearing impediment he has had since he was a child. He is a very smart man, but his life has been blocked by this handicap.

He would mispronounce words. He was known for getting names wrong. He would call 'Rosemary,' 'Margie' and it was often very embarrassing. Now, through our daily mentoring, we are at the point that he has begun giving speeches at my Toastmaster's Club. He is ready and willing to give a speech for the speech contest. Everybody is proud of him; me especially.

Shon knew and loved Josh, and he has met my parents. He met them when they came to Tulsa for Josh's Life Celebration service. He would always tell me my parents were like royalty. Queen Monique and King Robert. Shon is a good brother and a strong believer. He is familiar with my father's condition and we often speak about ideas for finding pathways of healing to help my father.

One idea I have has come from the stories of how St. Francis talked to the animals. Every day, a scissor-tailed flycatcher has been landing on my driveway or on the crepe myrtle tree by the curb. I tell this amazing bird he must be so full of the praises of God for how beautiful the Lord has made him.

Today, the bird arrives with his whole family and they land on the roof. The beautiful bird then flies down onto the driveway and standing there before me, opens and closes his striped wings three times. I am praising God for such a successful connection that the bird responds by showing off!

What if I can use this faith type of communication with my dad, and talk to him as if he can understand me? Would he respond?

My mom has invited me for Thanksgiving. I'm looking forward to flying to Orlando to visit my parents.

The relatively short flight feels more like a commute. I love flying and I am looking out of my window to see the beautiful white puffy clouds, and it feels like the glory of God is all around me.

"Welcome to Orlando International Airport," the flight attendant says as we land. I walk through the lobby, say "Hi!" to Mickey and Minnie Mouse, pass under the video of Sea World and take the escalator down to the baggage claim floor. My suitcase makes its way to me on the carousel; I gracefully find a space between my fellow travelers and lift it up and roll it through the sliding glass doors.

A rush of very warm, humid air immediately envelops me as I enter the busy and beautiful space around me. Orlando is a very different place than Tulsa.

My phone rings. It's my mom. She tells me that they are circling around and will be there soon and to be on the lookout for their champagne-colored Pontiac Bonneville. My idea of 'soon' is totally redefined as 50 minutes go by. While I am waiting, I become quite familiar with all the cars and people coming and going in what always feels like a tropical paradise, in sharp contrast to the changes of season in Tulsa.

When they finally pull up, I'm happy to see them. My mom gets out of the car to hug me while my dad remains seated on the passenger side.

"It's so good to have you with us again, Marc!" Mom says. It has only been two months since my last visit, but I'm taken aback by her lightweight frame and height. She still has her pretty long blonde hair. I want to give her a compliment; I tell her she looks good and she answers in her native French: "Je crois que j'ai pris un coup de vieux." I am not really sure what that means so I ask her and she says, 'prendre un coup de vieux' means 'taking a hit of old age.' What can I say? It's crowded, there are cars everywhere, so I load up the trunk and jump in the car.

My mom has planned for us to eat an early dinner at the airport Hyatt restaurant, so we drive around to the valet parking entrance, leave the car and take the elevator overlooking the airport lobby up to the fourth floor. Slowly, we make our way down the long hallways of the hotel and over to the restaurant.

We have a good lunch and everything seems to be going well until it is time to leave. On the way out we get distracted after paying the bill and lose sight of my father, who has somehow managed to wander down the big hotel hall.

We spot him standing quite far away, talking to a lady sitting at a desk. He is full of charm and waving his arms. My mom rushes off to the rescue and by the time she gets there, the lady is standing and looking seriously distressed. Upon reaching them, my mom manages to grab my dad while being vague and as to why my father is actually there, which only seems to raise more questions for the lady. This is all fresh to me, and from my removed viewpoint, my father looks so convincing in his approach and the lady so committed to helping him that I find their encounter to be humorous. Mainly, I see the difficulty for my mom, never knowing where or when my dad will go next, and the difficulty for my dad, who doesn't seem to realize what he is doing.

"That's why I always keep the front door of the apartment locked, so he can't ever leave without me knowing about it," my mother explains later. "Getting Dad back like this is not really the way I want to meet new people! We go out so little as it is. We used to go out together all the time."

That evening, I help Mom make the same delicious stuffing she made when we lived in France. Amongst other things, this involves peeling the rind off of tangerine skins, peeling the skin off boiling hot chestnuts and frying up chicken livers. After that, we set up the dining room table for the turkey dinner we are going to have the next day. Very early Thursday morning, I help her stuff the turkey and place it in the oven.

Thanksgiving is very animated. My brother, Greg comes over to the apartment in the mid-morning with his daughters, Jen and Elise, and his wife, Heather. They have flown in from Southern

California to be here and will be leaving the next day. Greg starts on the job of basting the turkey and stays working in the kitchen while chatting with Mom until it's time to serve the food.

My father chooses to sit near me in the living room. Heather, Jen, and Elise gather around the coffee table, sitting on a couch near us. Jen is in her twenties and running a business in Denver, Colorado, and Elise is getting ready to go to film school. They are extremely fond of their Grandmama and their Grandpapa, and recount with joy countless stories of their vacations spent together in Jackson Hole, Wyoming. Dad is listening contentedly and pitches in with affirming comments at key moments in their stories. He says: "That's right!" and "It was really great!"

Something good is happening because he seemingly has forgotten about "the equipment." At one point, a delightful outburst follows the announcement that we are going to eat soon and my father, standing before me, has much to say. I treat it like it is a normal conversation, and I encourage his talking, by giving him the best feedback I can, so he can feel welcome here, even though technically his words are compositions from a parallel universe.

It is a universe that I have been invited to travel with him. I can relate to him in this universe essentially because of the eye contact my father gives me. He still recognizes me and knows who I am. This eye contact is precious when it is present. When it is not present, I've been trying to establish a response from him to the sound of my voice — and talk to him like he can understand me, just like I've talked with the birds in Tulsa and they have responded to my voice.

My mom has brought out her best silverware, her best china, has candles lit on her silver candlesticks, and lovely placemats which rest upon a beautiful red tablecloth. We are all sitting somewhat formally, and eagerly enjoying the Thanksgiving feast.

My father is happy to be a part of this great culinary tradition and seems to be absorbing all the good cheer and fellowship being generated around him at this, *his* family table. He exclaims his pleasure: "That's wonderful!" and "You're right!" at choice times during the rhythm of the evening.

No one has really tried to start a conversation with my father, nor is anyone really saying *anything* to my father. My father doesn't seem to mind and is making the best of his time by attentively listening to each person's voice and diligently eating everything on his plate, right up to the last morsel of this tender, free-range turkey, specially-ordered from Williams-Sonoma in Winter Park.

When the evening is over, Greg, Heather, Jen and Elise wish us a good night and leave the apartment to go back to the airport Hyatt hotel. They walk down the balcony toward the elevator, waving goodbye and saying: "Goodbye Grandmama! Goodbye Grandpapa!"

They are sad to leave my mother, who has a special place in their hearts. My mother seems sad as well to see them go, as does my father. We come back into the kitchen and my mom speaks at length about how great it was to see her granddaughters, how happy Dad seemed to be, and how good the turkey was. Finally, she says how happy she is that Greg loaded up the dishwasher, and we don't have to do the dishes, and how thankful she is about the overall success of the evening.

Now that Thanksgiving is over, my mother has to once again face my father in the reality of his condition; that night, he urinates in their bed. Although my mother has placed several mats used for changing baby diapers under the sheets on his side of the bed, the bed gets wet. She wants me to go to the store and see if I can find an adult diaper for my dad that won't leak at night.

The following morning, I leave for the grocery store and come home with two different brands of adult diapers, which I artfully configure into one, hopefully, water-tight, super absorbent mighty adult diaper.

For the next few days of my one-week visit, I work on refining my so-called design to absorb more and leak less. I thought I would be helping — yes — but also be lightening the load in a celebratory way during this Thanksgiving week. I am already more involved with my dad's situation than I feel prepared for. Or am I more prepared than I think? The Lord seems to think I am.

MARC, CAN YOU STAY?

The next evening after Thanksgiving, around 11 p.m. Mom and I are getting ready to go to bed after sitting in the living room.

My dad is awake and wanders in. It is clear by his face that he needs a change of underwear as his underwear is very wet. I get out one of my newly beefed up, hopefully leak-proof adult diapers to put on him.

I take his hand and walk him into the bathroom.

He sits down on the toilet willingly.

"Dad, which leg is this?" I ask him, crouching by his right leg.

"Right leg," he says.

I say, "Very good. Please lift up your right leg."

He lifts it up. I put his foot through the underwear. "Now, Dad, which leg is this?" I ask him about his left leg which is next to the bathtub.

"Left leg," my father answers.

"That's right. Excellent. Please lift up your left leg."

He lifts it up. I put his foot through the underwear.

"Okay, we got it, Dad. Well done. You can stand up now."

He stands up and I pull up his underwear and then pull up his pajama pants. Dad tucks everything in his pants — his T-shirt and his pajama top — and then pulls the string tight and makes a good strong knot. I know his pajama top needs to be hanging loosely over his pants, but I am tired and let it go. I know my mother is tired as well.

I say: "Mom will be glad to see you." Then I give him a big hug which he is okay with, and he lifts his left arm and puts it over my shoulder. *Wow*! I'm thinking. *Affection from my dad!* This is a first.

Memories of physical affirmation from my father go back many years. I am not expecting him to reach out to me like this. Maybe it is because he is happy to see me again. He clearly sees me as his friend.

I cherish this moment, and it is a wonderful show of affection, and one of the few affectionate embraces that I remember him giving me.

We walk slowly out of the bathroom and then into the bedroom where his Monique helps him get back in bed.

She pulls up the sheets and says, "There! Now you are all snuggled under the covers."

My dad says, "Oh, this is so nice. Just what a bear needs. Now I can catch some fish!"

We smile and my mom asks me to sit down while she says a rather long prayer about asking the Lord to heal my father and protect the apartment. I say, "Amen," we hug and say, "Good night."

On Saturday morning, my mom comes into the guestroom where I am sleeping. From the look on her face, I know she has a very serious request.

"Marc, can you stay?" she asks me.

I am self-employed. I have my own auto detail business. I can reschedule customers when I need to.

So I say: "Sure, I can stay a little longer."

My mom seems okay with that answer. I know she has a doctor's appointment on Monday and they are concerned about what looks like a black lump on the X-rays, in her colon. She also asks me to pray for her, which I do at that moment and again during the weekend.

We have leftovers from the turkey dinner and dessert which we enjoy on Saturday and Sunday. I'm doing my best to be present to my dad, to talk with him and listen. My mom is taking a break to do some things for herself, now that I'm here with Dad.

I get Dad dressed in some of his elegant clothes and we take a walk on the balcony. The tropical climate here is sublime and very healing to my senses. I tell my dad that it is good to see him and because I am here, we can take walks on the balcony together.

Sunday night I feel good that my mom has had some time off. I am praying for my dad and have seen some response in him through smiles and nods of his head. I'm still riding high after spending almost 3 years helping my son Josh and writing the story of our amazing last days together before his death. He had been abused by his mother as a child, and by the grace of God, we had been able to heal, to walk out of that pain and to live a happy life.

Just at the point where he was most joyful and loving to be alive and to be with me, he died in his sleep at the age of 24. Nothing and nobody has been able to take his place. The only thing that gives me joy is to retell the stories of our amazing friendship by writing my book. It has just been published October 25, 2012, on Amazon and I am still very focused on promoting it.

Now, here I am at my mom and dad's house in Florida, with my father in his third year of Alzheimer's. I am concerned for my father and I am praying for a miracle healing in my mom's colon. I am visualizing the black mass in my mother's colon being dissolved by the living waters of the Holy Spirit and that area being filled with the light of Christ. Sunday night we spend more time praying for her to be healed.

Monday morning my mother drives herself to the doctor's appointment. She has not been able to do this in a long time because of needing to keep an eye on my dad.

After reviewing the new X-rays, the doctor tells my mother that he is still very concerned about her health. He wants to do more tests as there still seems to be a block in her colon.

That afternoon my mother comes into the guest room where I am sitting on one of the twin beds. She looks very concerned.

"Marc, can you stay?" she asks me.

I say, "You mean longer?"

My mother shakes her head. "No. I mean, can you stay?"

It is my mom asking me to stay, with a very serious look in her eyes.

I can see the wear on her face, and the toll that taking care of her Bobby these last three years has taken on her body. Now she is not only worrying about my father, but her own health is also in question.

"I am very concerned about this black spot on my colon. I don't feel as strong as I did before, Marc, to take care of Dad. I keep believing he can get better, but I'm tired of doing all this on my own. I feel weaker and it is scary. Can you stay?"

The request comes as a total surprise. Stay? For good? Live here?

If I do this, it will be a major life change. I can't possibly speak all my thoughts out loud right now. I am too busy thinking about the consequences and ramifications.

So, let me get this straight. You want me to give up my house in Tulsa, where I have lived for the past 25 years?

You want me to give up my auto detail business and my income that I've had for the last 25 years?

You want me to give up my friends from Toastmasters, my Church, give up taking care of my hundreds of customers and move to Florida where I don't know anybody and would have no source of income?

And you want me to give up promoting my book? And you want me to do all of this to take care of Dad?

My mother seems to actually hear all my reactions to her request, and just says: "Yes, could you, Marc?"

So, my next thoughts turn to my father. The sickness has changed his personality. I find him to be more of a friendly father than the dad I knew in previous years. But he also is much more out of touch with his world. He doesn't remember much. He can no longer read, except for a few words in big letters. And the biggest change is that he can no longer write.

This is a big loss for him because he loved to write. After graduating from Yale, he dreamed of becoming a writer. Financial constraints obliged him to take a sales position and he also decided to attend business school in the evenings.

During this time, he made notes about everything and kept the notes for years. The log book in which he wrote about our sailing trip to the British Virgin Islands in 1974 is right on a cart by the dinner table. I glance at the notes of everything he wrote. He kept meticulously detailed entries involving compass readings, distances, locations, map coordinates, the events of the day and readings of the stars at night.

Conversation is difficult now. When he talks, what he says makes little sense. It takes an act of love on my mom's part to engage with him, to hear him out and to respond.

He also wanders, as I have already seen after our lunch at the Hyatt restaurant. He has left the house a few times, but he has also walked out of a dentist appointment, summoning the Winter Park police to search for him. This turned out to be a great faith story — as an officer felt God had led him to find my dad sitting on a bench in front of the All Saints Episcopal Church.

My problem personally was that we had never been that close. Basically, I felt that my dad had been very disconnected from me after the age of 13, and had set me up in situations that could have destroyed me were it not for the saving grace of Jesus. He had taught me some cool things when I was a kid but when I needed him to be a father, most of the time he was traveling on business, and working late hours when he was home. So it was this, "hush, hush, your father is working" situation.

I felt that when it came down to it, he had just not been there for me. More than that, I felt he had messed up my life. So in that moment of decision, I'm dealing with a series of positive and negative feelings all rapidly piling up before me.

But it isn't just about my dad. It is about my mom asking me this question, asking me to help her. I cannot say 'no' to my mother. That's what my mom is saying: "Yes, can you? I mean I will take care of your financial needs."

If I were married and had young children at this point in my life and had to be overseeing my business, the answer would've been: "Mom, I have a family to take care of and a business to run. I will come over like I have been, every seven weeks, and help with Dad."

But I am living alone. My beloved son, my best friend, went to be with his Heavenly Father on March 19, 2010. My ex-wife is long gone, since June of 2008, and that relationship is over.

Did I think it through? Not really. Did I realize what I was getting myself into? Not a chance. Did I negotiate some kind of deal financially? This is my whole life we are talking about, and I am turning 55 very soon.

As I look back, I wish I had sat down with my mom to count the costs. But in the present, it is just a verbal agreement based on goodwill. I take time to pray about it and I feel God's grace settling in me with a sense of peace. The Lord is saying, "Stay."

So I tell my mom: "I will stay."

ALL HEROES PLEASE STAND UP

I am sleeping well at night. I am in Florida and by the grace of God, I am willing to let go of the life that I have known. I have to let go of promoting my book to be here with my parents. I have to give up my house to live in their 'computer room.'

This room is furnished with two twin beds and a desk that is part of a bookshelf upon which the computer sits. Next to the shelf-desk is a three-drawer dresser with a lamp and a printer on it, and on the side next to the bed is a very wide closet, filled with my mom and dad's clothes.

It's hard for my mom. She wants to keep everything the way it was before my dad changed, though my presence here means making room for me. For his part, my dad does not seem to have the slightest attachment to anything in this room.

Despite my new living space reduction, I still find God with me. Daily I am praying for my mom, and concentrating my focus on finding pathways of healing for my dad, which is what I am here for.

Fortunately, I have already put some preparation into this situation by making a short movie for my Tulsa Toastmasters' Club addressing the essential elements needed to find pathways of healing for my dad. In the film, I conclude the following:

- ✓ **Non-Literal Interpretation is the way of listening to his language.**
- ✓ **Creative insight is needed to respond.**

✓ **Interaction is a Hands-On Experience where my Personal Presence Level is equal to Jesus's Presence Level.**
  ✓ **New Pathways can be found to bring healing.**

I feel that I am on a mission to improve my dad's situation enough that it will once again make a close relationship possible between my mom and my dad. Thus, my dad would be reconnected enough with my mom that she could handle taking care of him. They could work things out together, and I could go back to my house in Tulsa.

But this hope turns out to be very unrealistic. I'm still underestimating my dad's progress. He is soon going to be entering the dreaded anger period, which happens after an acute onset of the disease and is known to be a breaking point for many families because the patient becomes violent and defiant.

Many say: "Time to get help. It's become too demanding. I can't keep working and taking care of him. A nursing home? Assisted living? Let's look into those options now."

Those kinds of decisions sometimes send the afflicted one over the edge. I do not want that to happen to my dad. Neither does my mom. Losing the familiarity of his environment would be a shock to my father's system; like hypothermia, where the water is too cold for the body to recover.

I have heard from my nurse friend working with Alzheimer patients that once the disease is already present in the patient, a sudden, unexpected, emotional shock, caused by an event which seems overwhelmingly difficult to deal with, will trigger an acute onset of Alzheimer's.

So if one traumatic experience can trigger an acute onset of Alzheimer's, a second traumatic experience can mark the point of no return once the disease is advanced.

Finding out exactly just what was the traumatic experience that brought the onset of my dad's condition is definitely on my agenda.

I am not sure that my mom knows, and I pray that it will somehow come to light during our conversation.

My dad's needs are constant. They are so demanding at times that I really cannot even take care of something as precious to me as my book. *The Coolness of Josh* has just been published on Amazon. After 32 months of writing and covering the many details of this creative process, it is really great seeing my book on Amazon.

It is one of those momentous achievements of a lifetime.

That is until you say, 'How momentous?'

My book ranks 3,544,285 on Amazon and is not yet selling.

Is coming to Florida, for Thanksgiving for a week, just a little time off from me marketing my book? Wrong! It is a lot of time off! Now I have to put my book on the back burner.

With the time I have, I am working with Elaine, my genius format lady, to make the e-book version for Kindle. Besides this, I have little time to ask friends for reviews of the book on Amazon or to promote it. The evening of December 23, I text Josh's favorite teacher and mentor, Charles Burris, and write: *Hey Charles, my book is published on Amazon.com.*

On Christmas Eve morning, I cut out a skirt from wrapping paper to put under the newly arrived Christmas tree. My mother and I assemble an assortment of presents on the skirt under the tree. We have some ornaments and I bought some multi-colored lights from the local hardware store.

We have a tree, thanks to my brother's initiative. L.L. Bean has always been big with my mom, and staying true to the family tradition, Greg ordered a Christmas tree, which was shipped, freshly cut, from Maine to the Swift doorstep.

Of course, I would have loved some time off to hunt for a tree. There are many tents filled with trees that I pass on my way to shop for food at Whole Foods and the local grocery store. I am also aware that providing the tree enables Greg to have a part in Mom and

Dad's Christmas. Greg will not be here for Christmas since he is very involved with his work and his own family.

My mom longs to go to Mass at St. Margaret Mary's Catholic Church, but it has become confusing for my dad to take communion, as well as to stay in the pew in church. She does not want to go without him, and would rather stay home. We do our best to relive the Christmas story, reading the accounts of Luke and Matthew. I also put into action my DJ skills from the time I was a DJ at Brown University. I play CDs of time-honored Christmas Carols, a tradition that goes back to my parent's years living in Paris, France.

My parents have recently bought CD versions of those classic albums and it is a joy to hear those carols again. We listen to songs about that night when Jesus was born and when the shepherds heard angels singing and saw the heavenly Glory shining all around them.

"Glory to God in the highest,
    And on earth peace, goodwill toward men!" (Luke 2:14 NKJ).

CHRISTMAS EVE

It is Christmas Eve dinner time. My father kicks off the evening's conversation as we sit at the dining room table, this Friday night. Holding our forks and knives about to dig in, my father says: "Where are we driving to?"

Does this prompt hysterical laughter? It certainly could have. The joy level is still high from our celebration preparations and if we had started laughing, my father would have picked up on it, and laughed that knowing laugh, as if he had set out to say something funny, and he was glad that we were catching on.

The reason I think that hysterical laughter did not ensue, was that we had spent the previous twenty minutes trying to get him to sit down. He repeated many antics — from sitting in my mother's chair to lifting up his chair and moving it, to standing with his leg poised over the chair but never actually *sitting down*, to trying to remove the cushion from his chair — all the while saying: "Like this? *Like this?*"

Given the increased frustration level my mother and I are feeling, by the time my father finally does sit down, we are not amused.

It is an effort to keep being kind and patient, and not lose it, which would have expressed itself through those &%#! symbols characters use in comic books. His remark is still challenging enough to make it interesting, but the idea of driving somewhere means leaving *to go* there.

Instead of a ha-ha moment, the overriding feeling is that my mother and I are very set on my father staying right there, in his chair. We keep an eye on him and remain focused, with serious-looking faces, until we can relax a little bit and lighten up enough to trust that he will stay put.

It's now time to respond to the 'question.' To answer this question literally would be both too difficult, and too downright serious.

Literal interpretation and legalism are in a serious business practice together. The problem with people who have Alzheimer's is that they seriously practice making fun of legalists and run circles around the literal.

Having learned that, my mother and I are not going to say, "Bob, you are in the *dining room* now. You are not in *a car*. We're having dinner now. This is *your house.*"

He was not just waking up after surgery. He was not lying in a hospital bed with a nurse leaning over him saying: "*Hello, Bob.* Can you tell me *where you are?*"

The reason this was funny to me was that I myself had been in a similar situation in 1977 in New York City, at Lenox Hill Hospital. I was waking up after brain surgery. My life had gotten pretty messed up and there I was at 19 being told I had a tumor the size of a baseball in my head.

Thanks to my mom's Sunday school placement of me with two nuns, I knew about Jesus and I had called upon Him and put my life in His care. Waking up from the surgery, I heard a nurse talking to an elderly lady, saying: "Do you know where you are?" I was astonished to hear her answer: "Yes, I'm in the 42nd St. subway station."

I felt pretty good waking up and I knew exactly where I was. I determined to make the most of a golden opportunity for humor. When the same nurse came over to me and leaned over to make sure I heard her, she asked me: "Marc, can you tell me where you are?" I was determined to say something funny, outrageous even,

I'm sure, but had no set answer. What blurted out of my mouth was as much of a surprise to her as it was a delight to me.

"Yes. Tokyo!"

The nurse did not laugh nor did she correct me. She just gave me some kind of sly look while I chuckled inwardly.

I was quite comfortable with these kinds of situations like: "where are we driving to?" and actually enjoyed the challenge of finding ways to go deeper through what I termed a 'non-literal interpretation.' I had a history of true stories, most of them humorous, based on giving creative answers to such questions.

We say grace and are eating which makes me think of one such story of a meal during a Catholic Charismatic summer retreat in San Antonio, Texas. We regularly ate at the same table in the dining room with the same group of people. A priest, Father Luke, was part of our group, and he felt, of course, that it was always up to him to say grace.

On this particular day, he was late in coming and we were all very ready to eat. So someone said: "Marc, why don't you say grace?"

I was more than happy to do so. I made a short prayer thanking God for the food and for our time together. There was a shared "amen!" and just as we were picking up our silverware to begin eating lunch, Father Luke arrived at our table somewhat out of breath, sat down and said: "Sorry I'm late." Then lifting up his right hand to his forehead he said: "In the name of the Father and of the Son and of the Holy Spirit," and proceeded to say grace. He assumed we had all been waiting for him to say grace so we could begin. We obliged him and went along with his prayer.

After finishing he looked up with a big smile, ready to eat and saw that everyone was looking at him kind of funny. "Am I missing something?" he asked, looking a little embarrassed.

One of the ladies said: "Well Father, you see, Marc already said grace." Father Luke then started to process the fact that we had not felt it necessary to wait for him and said: "Oh, I didn't realize."

Everyone started to feel uncomfortable. At this point, it felt like the ball was definitely in my court since I had said the first grace. I thought about what I could say to ease the tension and what came to mind were the teachings of the past week, which had been focused on the power of praise and worship. The saying we had heard several times was: "He who sings, prays twice."

Armed with some verbal acuity, I reached out my hand toward Father Luke, who was facing me, and said, with great flourish,

"Father, it's OK! He who prays twice, *sings!*"

He burst out laughing, as did the whole table. Our meal went on with merriment.

After dinner, my father, no doubt inspired by the Christmas carols and the green, red, blue and orange lights on the tree, is very willing to get up and walk over to the couch in the middle of the room. He sits down on the side closest to the tree, and my mother takes her place next to him. He stretches out, propping his legs up on the coffee table wearing his blue leather slippers on his feet.

He is enjoying the colors of the lights and ornaments on the tree as my mom hands him a Christmas gift. He spends a long time appreciating the wrapping paper on the gift, laughing and saying affirmative remarks such as: "Well, isn't that something!" and "That's great!" We open Christmas presents and Dad is in top shape, enjoying the festivities and happily sitting next to his Monique.

CELEBRATING AT THE TABLE

On Christmas morning, I go online and see that Charles Burris must have purchased my book and had it overnighted to his home because right there on Amazon is the most brilliant review from him. Once I read Charles Burris's review, it immediately becomes apparent that this far outweighs any and all of the reviews my friends could have possibly ever written, even if I had paid them *large* sums of money to do so. I had to let go of promoting my book and now here is a review from Josh's favorite teacher and mentor.

I am in awe of what God has done for me.

During the many difficult nights when I feel more like I am living out a Franciscan vow of poverty, the Lord has been saying: "Trust me." He also says: "Stay here. You will find joy and happiness and prosperity in this place." I do my best to trust him.

Now, on this Christmas Day, a little over one month after I traveled to Florida for a short vacation, I sit gaping at the computer screen, marveling at this five-star review. I have the utmost respect for Charles Burris. He is a passionate teacher and writer with enormous political and historical insight. His generous review is a huge compliment to me and a personal endorsement of my book:

> "He was my favorite high school student in a 20+ year teaching career. He was a brilliant writer and engaging conversationalist, always celebrating life and pursuing the elusive search for its deeper meaning. Marc Swift's

poignant and moving memoir of the loss of his son and the celebration of his life is perfectly named. For Josh was indeed "cool." He was one of the most amazing persons I have ever known. Josh was also a master at concealing some of the darker secrets that had tragically shaped his wonderful life. Marc candidly explores these mysteries and reveals their horrific nature. Two aphorisms of the philosopher Friedrich Nietzsche captures this "coolness" of Josh: "That which does not kill us makes us stronger," and "He who would learn to fly one day must first learn to stand and walk and run and climb and dance; one cannot fly into flying." While in his time on Earth, Josh danced and soared high above his fellow groundlings. He is deeply missed but never forgotten by those of us who had the treasured experience of knowing him. Celebrate his wonderful memory by reading this insightful and very unique memoir. For then you too will know of 'the coolness of Josh.'"

~ Charles Burris

My mom comes by and I share with her the good news: "Burris (that's what Josh called him) wrote a review!"

"What an amazing review! It is the kind of thing you are still in awe of in 10 years," she says. "It is something you will never forget!"

This happy event leads to some tenderness and softening of my situation. Celebration is in order for the next few days.

My mom says, "Why don't you read your book to Dad? You know he wants to hear it! He can't say that to you, but he can hear you read it."

She's right. So I sit my father down in his favorite brown leather chair and make sure he is comfortable. I sit down on the white couch by the back windows and pick up my book.

"Dad, this is the book I wrote, *The Coolness of Josh*," I tell him.

Starting from the first chapter, I read him all the words that I have lovingly crafted and that mean so much to me. His eyes are open. He nods his head every now and then. He takes it in, this gift from his son and it finds a welcome home in his heart.

He hears my book one section at a time. We take the journey together during that week between Christmas and New Year's Day. I feel guilty that I should be reading him Scriptures, but I know this is God, God in *me* for him to hear what I have written. To my great surprise, it is also God speaking through him, for me to hear, which utterly surprises me.

My father is mostly nodding, but picks up his head and listens more intently, as I finish reading this passage:

> *It was as though Josh left me a note in my own native heart language saying, "It is going to happen, it really will happen one day. I will see you again. Soon. A bientôt Papa!"*

After reading, 'it really will happen one day,' my father speaks up for the first time: "That's right!"

Then after, 'I will see you again. Soon. A bientôt Papa!' he says: "You're onto something really big!"

When we get to the end of the book, my dad looks at me with one of his reassuring smiles, his eyes half closed, and he says: "Very good. Well done!"

He actually can affirm me as if everything is normal.

That evening we are happily seated at the dining room table. Celebrating Christmas means having fun. I am thinking about the good food and the restaurants where we have gone in the past.

"Mom, if you owned a restaurant what would you call it?"

"*Chez Les Bons Vivants*," my mother answers in French, with ease and right away. It means: "With those who have a love for living and enjoy life."

It sounds like just the kind of place where I would have been right at home, laughing, with good food and happy hearts, glad to be with each other: the happy feast.

I grew up with an image of a long table with a happy family eating, in France, with open windows overlooking a beautiful garden. That was always my ultimate dream — the Sunday lunch table, laid out for a sumptuous feast with family and friends laughing and celebrating life, in the warm French countryside, surrounded by the soft breeze, awakened by the sweet smell of lavender. I can relax at the dining room table with this idea and have fun.

To complement the Christmas tree, lit up with the Christmas lights a little further back in the living room, we have decided to have candles on the table. My parents have collected a variety of candleholders over the years, so I make it my job to set up seven or eight candles.

I use some long matches to light the candles and watch the burning flames soften and melt the wax of different colors. They each have a variety of fragrances. I gather this happy assortment of candles before me and love watching all their glowing flames. These candles are my little flock that I can move around each night and arrange in different patterns.

My father is engrossed in making his own patterns, folding his napkin diagonally, then in half, exploring various geometrical designs, after which he leans back in his chair to contemplate his work. "Umm, hum," I hear him say in appreciation. I think the current mental state of my father must be contagious because here I am making layout designs for the candle holders and getting into it.

Time for a story. I ask my mom about the marvelous, magical wonderland where they lived in France. It was a remarkable French estate, the large house surrounded by a moat, through which flowed a river full of fish, with a stone bridge crossing the river and leading up the path to the *rez de chausse* of the busy residence.

The road for automobiles, after entering the main gate, split to the left and to the right and headed upward, around the circumference of this lovely land, and took the cars around to the back of the house where there was the main entrance.

Facing outward from the back was a world of happy well-being. Chickens and goats could be seen, the daily spoils of hunting and fishing were being prepared, cows rummaged on the pastureland of the dairy farm, which produced eggs and milk each morning, and a quaint vineyard was nestled behind a greenhouse filled with orange trees and lemon trees.

The road in the back led off to the left toward a bridge which crossed *la Saune*, a sandy banked river where Francoise — my mom's mother — was fond of spending her time during the heat of the summer.

The big house and the surrounding area were called, "Cillery."

At the table, my dad is eating and enjoying his meal, which this evening is chicken pieces cut from a rotisserie chicken that I bought at Whole Foods, served with green beans and rice. This is a meal that is particularly suited to my mother's cooking style and we eat it often.

I have been to Cillery once, at the tender age of six years old. I can remember sensing that it was a magical place, but there was much I had not been able to explore.

"It seems like it was such a magical place. The children must've loved it!" I say to my mom.

"Oh, you have no idea! My sister Helen's children, Catherine, Christian, Anne, Philippe and Elise, really loved it. You have no idea how they loved it! To them, it was really a wonderful place. When they heard that it was going to have to be sold, they were in such a state. They said, 'We will save our money, we will buy it.' They could not imagine no longer being there."

"I believe you, Mom," I say. "I would have done the same thing: anything to hold on to it."

"You know children," she says. "They like a place, they feel like it's their home and then all of a sudden...It's gone."

My mother's comment strikes a chord in me. "Yeah. It hurts. As a child in such a place of wonder, you think it will be there forever. When you lose something like that, you can spend the rest of your life trying to get it back."

I think of a book that Dad gave me.

"Dad gave me a French book called *Le Grand Maulnes*. It was about a boy who discovers this wonderful, magical place, with gardens and a chateau one day when he is out walking on a country road. He falls in love with a beautiful lady he sees and the experience changes his whole life. He comes back home in wonder at it all. Of course, the next day all he can think about is going back there, but he can't figure out how he got there. He thought it would come to him naturally, but the path eludes him."

I pause. Then I look over at my mom. "Somehow, on some level, this must be what Dad is feeling; trying to get back to this magical place, gardens and château, the best part of his life."

On this night, my father is taking his time eating, expressing his enjoyment of the story with affirming outbursts, and though I am expecting my mom to respond to me, it is my dad who answers with a resounding: "That's right!"

My father is finishing his supper, bearing his fork down on top of even the last kernel of rice on his plate. He has impeccable table manners and he maintains them consistently, to the delight of my mother.

I'm not sure whether my mother understands the full ramifications of what my father has just said. *Does his timely exclamation confirm that he is trying to get back to the best part of his life?* Either way, Dad seems happy and Mom continues with her story: "And then there were so many flowers, there was a whole flower garden. I enjoyed making 'des bouquets'. Arrangements, that's a big word, but you know flowers in vases. It was important to have flowers."

I did most of the shopping during that time with them and I did my best to bring back flowers as often as I could for my mom. She would carefully shorten the stem of each rose over the kitchen sink, lift each one under the cold running water after cutting it and then arrange it in one of her crystal vases, a third filled with water.

We would all enjoy the flowers until they started to wane. Then it was time for me to get more. Having these well-loved flowers, beautifully displayed in their vase, on the living room table, gave us all reason for a cheerful outlook; keeping them around became a pleasurable discipline for me.

HOPE FOR HEALING?

The following week my father has an appointment to see the doctor. We make the laboriously slow trek with my dad, leading him across from the fifth-floor apartment on the balcony to the elevator. It must be said that the view from this Winter Park, Florida balcony is breathtaking, with Florence, Italy, style red tiles on the house tops and magnificent villas and their glistening swimming pools, kitty-corner to the tall wooden fence lined with ever growing trees filled with tropical green foliage behind the long line of parked luxury cars.

Right by the elevator are three beautiful palm trees always poised with grace and style to welcome us. It is with a mixture of feelings that I am walking with my father, both enjoying the beauty of this tropical resort and feeling the pain of my father's difficulties.

We move into the elevator, press the first-floor button and wait. We feel suspended for a minute in this elevator that was the beginning of so many dinner outings to Brio's, my mother and father's favorite posh Italian restaurant.

The elevator door opens and my mother goes first and the three of us walk slowly toward the car. I am holding my father's hand. We cross the driveway which is the only road coming down the center of this Spanish-styled stucco apartment complex, with red roofed covered parking on both sides.

We make it to the car, backed into their reserved space by my mother on return from their last outing. I open the passenger door for my father to sit down, and my father moves to his left and wants to sit in the back seat. In this slow process, much patience is needed.

After some encouraging words, he agrees to bend down and slides onto the front seat. My mother sits in the driver seat and I sit behind my father in the back seat.

By the time the three of us sit in the car, we are already showing signs of wear, so when we finally arrive at the doctor's office and sit down in the examination room, we are all quite tired.

However, I am soon to jarred out of any sense of rest as I come face to face with my father's neurologist and with the maddening realization that our society's medical world is very happy to simply *manage* Alzheimer's. To simply manage Alzheimer's along its course to destruction.

My dad's neurologist looks at me like I am insulting his profession when I suggest that my dad might be able to receive healing and make "progress."

"No, no! Not a chance! It's even much too late for him to receive any medication that could help," the doctor says.

"I am determined to make progress," I tell him. "I believe Jesus can heal him."

"There's nothing to support that medically in all I've read. Don't kid yourself, Bob has Dementia and it is just going to play itself out."

Both my mom and I are taken aback by the word 'Dementia,' each of us for different reasons. My mom's attitude is that her Bob is suffering from 'memory loss.' She is unwilling to use the word, 'Alzheimer's' with either her family or her neighbors. To add to my father's condition with a second diagnosis like 'Dementia' is too much for her to handle.

For my part, I have learned a lot about the Alzheimer's disease from a girl I made friends with who worked nine hours a day with Alzheimer patients. I also had a customer in Tulsa for many years who had Dementia and started acting crazy and I don't see my dad acting this way.

Although technically, both diseases overlap and have elements in common, the neurologist does regard my father as an Alzheimer's patient primarily and realizes this may have been a faux pas on his part.

"Okay, 'Alzheimer's,' if that's what you want to call it," he says.

After that confrontation, he is very careful to only use the word *Alzheimer's*. This episode leaves me feeling even less reassured of the doctor's competence, and of the competence of the medical world as they assign 'scientifically' precise labels for these diseases, yet can make unintelligent general statements like, "It is too late in the progression of the disease for us to do anything that could help him."

At this point, let us briefly review a healing ministry's definition of what is going on during the course of the Alzheimer Disease. The author, Joan Hunter, is the daughter of Charles and Frances Hunter, who are famous for their healing ministry:

> "Alzheimer's Disease is characterized by a progressive loss of mental function. Part of the brain degenerates, destroying nerve cells which can no longer transmit signals from the brain to the body. This severely debilitating condition can lead to the person requiring constant supervision and becoming totally dependent, for all activities of daily living, upon another person. The total disorientation, personality changes, abnormal behavior, and loss of memory affect the person as well as the entire family."

> Joan Hunter. *Healing the Whole Man Handbook.*
> Whitaker House, Copyright 2005.

It is a real disappointment, after all of my previous efforts, not to hear any words of hope from the doctor, and to be told there will be no signs of improvement.

I have prayed thus far, with expectant faith.

I keep praying for his brain to heal, day after day, and after each round of prayer, there follows a day of no apparent change.

There are several good volumes written about the plaque, and the neurotransmitters and the nefarious onset and progress of the disease called Alzheimer's.

I make no claim to presenting a "comprehensive" approach to the problem, especially since, as far as my father is concerned, all the knowledge in the world has only availed my father an outing to the doctor's office and — besides another bill — another letdown.

At this point, there is doubt and I ask myself this question: *Is the neurologist right? Is it too late?*

But deep down *I know* there is more and that it is not too late. From my point of view, the neurologist is being too learned and too rational, and too sure that a pharmaceutically-based management solution is the answer.

I want to tell the good doctor what Hamlet says to Horatio:

"There are more things in heaven and earth, Horatio
Than are dreamt of in your philosophy."
            Hamlet, Act 1, Scene 5. William Shakespeare.

KID MARC

After long, frustrating weeks of prayer for my father's brain, I still am only reaching him in small ways. All my preconceived ideas, all my methods, even all my hopes have become seriously challenged.

I am not just here *to manage* this disease in him. The management and care taking part is something I can do, but it is not my main line purpose for my life.

My purpose here is to connect with my dad and to improve his situation. With my auto detail business in Tulsa, I detailed over 12,000 cars during a period of 25 years. I wasn't happy just 'cleaning' these cars. To me, the point was that I was improving these cars. I stayed in business for 25 years by saying to customers, "I can make your car look new again," and the customers demonstrated over and over that I was right. "Wow, it does look new again." Some added, "It looks even better than the day I bought it!"

So here in Florida, I am still the same guy. Just because I feel like I am an oversized guy trying to live in a dwarf's house does not change anything. My heart still sees that I have a mission to find pathways of healing for my dad and I believe this mission is from God. I expect to make a difference. Otherwise why give up everything for this job?

I believe that if Jesus Himself comes here in person and if He only says the Word, my dad will be healed and restored to the fullness of health.

I believe that it is God Himself who "gives life to the dead and calls those things which do not exist as though they did." (Romans 4: 17 NKJ).

I also believe that Jesus is interested in healing the whole man, and that is a process, and a process takes time. There is a reason my father got Alzheimer's and not Parkinson's disease, or Lou Gehrig's disease or a stroke, or cancer, or M. S., or a heart attack.

My spiritual father, T.L. Osborn, used to say: "We are God's hands and God's feet. God is counting on us to do His work." Perhaps, it *is* about personal presence, in a down-to-earth way. Being at the place where he is at, my mother and I can enable him to find new life within himself. I do not realize at this moment that I, too, will find new life within me.

After so many laborious sessions, there is one thing I do know: that it isn't about putting my hand on my father's head and praying for the reconnection in my dad's brain of his neurotransmitters, or his neural pathways, or his neuro-receivers.

Even though, scientifically, all the elements are now in need of repair as far as his brain is concerned, trying to heal his brain head on — no pun intended — isn't the way to do the repair job.

My mother also believes her Bob can be healed. After all, he did jail ministry for fifteen years in Orlando. (My mother did jail ministry for ten years.) The Lord was with him, was he not?

Filled with that hope, she took my dad earlier in September on the somewhat difficult journey of riding the train to Jacksonville to attend Francis MacNutt's *School of Healing Prayer*. At the school, they told her that they were not satisfied with the results of using prayer for the healing of Alzheimer's.

"We have had limited results. Caring presence, repetition, and other methods must be needed in addition to praying," the Prayer Team leaders informed her, adding that: "Someone who knows and cares for the patient personally might be able to bring about healing, and see their prayers answered. Remember the scripture in John 15: 13: "I demand that you love each other as much as I love you. And here is how to measure it; the greatest love is shown when a person lays down his life for his friends." (TLB).

Like the glimmer of the first dawn decisively dispels the night, I hear the voice of my inner child, decidedly breaking the silence.

My inner child speaks louder each day. This voice comes from a little kid, pulling on my sleeve, trying to get my attention.

One day after another round of prayer for the healing of my father's neuro-pathways, I say "Amen," and then I hear his voice speaking clearly to me.

"Isn't his brain the reason he got into this jam to start with?" he says.

When I look down, I can see and hear *me* — young Marc, an eight-year-old kid.

"Yeah, man!" I respond with enthusiasm, so glad to be talking with my new friend. "Dad was *always* living out of his brain."

"To the detriment of his caring and compassion, like toward me for instance," young Marc responds.

"You're right!" I say. "I'm so glad you're here. But where did you come from?"

"I figured I'd lend a hand with Dad, you know, as an answer to prayer since you've been praying so much for him to be healed," he says. "It was so painful back then. Do you remember on winter vacation in the Swiss Alps, going up the cog railway from Wengen to Kleine Sheidegg, to the foot of the Eiger, sitting across from Dad? He was looking very absorbed and in thought."

"Yeah!" I say.

"I was so excited about skiing and he was somewhere else, in his own think tank. 'A bomb blew up an ambassador's car in broad daylight,' he said after a while. I said something back and he said,

'Yeah, still.' That was it, our vacation bonding-talk for the half hour we sat facing each other."

"Yeah, I remember," I say. "He did not seem happy."

"Exactly," young Marc says. "So what good would it do, to just get all that brain stuff going again?"

"I totally agree! It would not do much good. That's a good point," I say. "It is a welcome relief to admit it. Maybe Dad is still trying to go to that once familiar place himself. Maybe he is still in the habit of finding answers there in that brain space, and he doesn't know about the new management, which simply mocks his attempts?"

"Which simply mocks his attempts is right," young Marc says. "What a cruel mockery for a man used to solving problems for large corporations, such as Deutsche Shell, the Belgian government, and Renault, to still be going there. He can't even play tic-tac-toe. He cannot complete a simple O or an X in the grid. You still have the drawing."

"In fact 'cruel mockery' does play a big part in this equation," I respond to my younger self. "It challenges me. Mockery was part of my upbringing, I saw my own father mock others."

"Yes, I remember. It was painful," says young Marc.

"That is why I think, it is essential to never, never give into that ugly attitude again," I say. "We must make positive statements only, and stand strong against the daily temptations to ridicule him back when he looks ridiculous, or to say a flippant comment. What do you think, young Marc?"

"To be positive, would be good," he answers pensively. "So, if we are combating a spirit of mockery and the healing of his brain is not yet happening, is there another way to reach him before he becomes totally out of touch?"

"This is like talking with me as a kid!" I say.

"Call me kid Marc," he says. "We have to figure this stuff out."

It is after a moment of silence that I hear kid Marc's magical voice again.

"It's simple," he says.

"Go ahead, my young friend Marc. I'm all ears."

"You remember growing up and hearing all about the communist regime in Russia, and hearing about Stalin's dictatorship. It's like Dad is under the power of a ruthless dictatorship and we need a revolution to get him out of there."

Kid Marc is right. I remember how smart I was at eight.

"Power to the people! Power back to Bob!" I answer him. "A revolution is needed!"

"A revolution to stop the tyrannical rule of the Alzheimer's dictatorship over Dad. Power back to Bob!" says kid Marc.

"So what is the lie that is going down in our father that is making the claim to dictatorship?"

It isn't long before I hear the voice of kid Marc exclaiming: "That his brain is King!"

"That his brain is King. Right on my friend," I answer him. "He has used his brain for everything — to understand, to comprehend, to analyze, to determine, to make decisions, to guide, to evaluate, to judge, to communicate, to plan, to relate. It's how he planned his whole life. It's a life-long habit."

Kid Marc: "We'll have to start a new habit in him to depose the dictator!"

"Indeed. A new habit. So what's the plan?" I say.

"We'll need to find a way to outsmart the brain. We need to circumvent his brain since everything going into it reaches a dead end."

"Dead end is right! This is a really bad deal," I say louder than normal.

"Are you okay, Marc?" asks my mom from the kitchen, overhearing my shout.

"Yeah, Mom, thanks. I'm fine. Just talking back to some jerk on the phone," I answer.

Kid Marc says, "There must be some way to undermine this dominating tyrant!"

"Yeah, we have to stop that tyrant! How do oppressed people overrule dictatorships?" I ask.

Kid Marc asks me "Can you find out? Check it out."

"Yeah, sure. I'm sure it's simple," I say.

OUTSMARTING THE BRAIN

Feeling a sense of urgency, I apply my spare time for a few nights to research the tactics, mindsets and methods for liberation used by those dispossessed people in history who were oppressed by dictators.

The violent methods are obviously *not the way* to fight in this situation.

It must be emphasized how often 'nonviolent' methods have been successful in history. 'Nonviolence' does not mean wimpy, passive, submissive or 'nice.' On the contrary, the strength of spirit and body, wisdom and mental resolve are all the more required, because it still is a confrontation. Sharp in word and action, yes; just not a fight in the streets with mortar, tanks, and tear gas — hence the word, 'nonviolent.'

I look into the science of political struggle for help with my strategy. How are revolutions against dictators accomplished? How do I go from the dictatorship of his sickness to the liberation of his (even if limited) well-being?

Historically the shift in power is from a dictatorship to a democracy. The term — democratic — though it has been misused and confused, is associated with a confirmation of the worth of individuals, civil rights and liberties, free expression of opinions, alternative candidates and decisions marked by a majority vote, with the leadership that best leads and represents the people.

The term *dictatorship* is associated with a person or a group claiming *the right* to rule the government system and society, without regard for constitutional limits or interest in elections to select officials representing the population. In a dictatorship, civil liberties are non-existent and opposition is taken care of by repression.*

In order to combat this dictatorship trying to rule my father, I have made a definition of 'dictatorship' in terms of my father's situation. The definition of 'dictatorship':

"DICTATORSHIP: *A stronghold ruled by martial law established upon the total control of absolute despotism."* *

In the medical mindset of our Western civilization of the 20-21ˢᵗ centuries, it is technically classified as a 'Disease' named 'Alzheimer's.' In a Venetian diagram of overlapping similarities, some neurologists support the view that it can also be separate/integral with a 'Disease' named 'Dementia.' Both classifications equally reveal a ruthless dictatorship in the pursuit of an inhuman goal.

Using the language of power struggles, I have defined the dictatorship's goals for my father. The definition of the 'dictatorship's goals':

THE ALZHEIMER'S DISEASE-DICTATORSHIP'S GOALS:

1. *To reduce and ultimately annihilate all relationship connections of recognition, communication, affection and love between the democrat and his loved ones.*
2. *To isolate the democrat and his or her loved ones.*
3. *To leave both parties separated, isolated and alienated.*

Thus, all confrontation with the dictatorship on the democrat's part is done by means of *nonviolent defiance.*

The right to act in defiance is based on the *illegitimate* taking of power by the dictator and his subsequent rule by the use of repression and denial of all civil liberties.

Therefore, the right and purpose *to act* in nonviolent defiance begins with:

1. *"A denial of legitimacy to the dictator and a noncooperation with the regime."* *
2. *"A refusal to accept that the outcome will be decided by the means of fighting chosen by the dictatorship."* *

The goals in the nonviolent struggle for democracy are achieved in the following ways:

1. *"By progressively growing a 'democratic space,' by methodically building an independent society outside of the dictatorship's control."* *
2. *"By the use of 'nonviolent coercion.' Although the opponents' leaders remain in their positions and keep faith with their original goals, their ability to act is effectively being taken away from them."* *

I have to reset my mindset as a result of these studies. I realize that I have been sort of fighting his sickness and that by focusing on his sickness, even to heal it, I am dealing with it on its own terms.

*All references: Sharp, Gene. *From Dictatorship to Democracy*, The Albert Einstein Institute. 2002

THE RESISTANCE

I resolve that, from now on, I will face my dad as someone struggling 'in defiance of illegitimate powers' trying to control him.

The 'resistance' of the allied forces against the Nazis in World War II had been prominent in my upbringing in France during the 60's. My grandfather had been a war hero in both World Wars, and in World War II he had refused to cooperate with the government of Vichy, which, under Marechal Petain, had surrendered to the Germans.

My grandfather, Henri Barbet, set up his own underground network through the mountains into Spain and on to North Africa to aid young French men escape from being taken to the German labor camps. In fact, along with Cillery, my mother often talked at the dinner table about their perilous times in Lyon and the heroism of her father and how God had saved his life in the most miraculous way.

I'm sure being raised on the side of the resistance, rather than on the side of the oppressor, helped me enormously. I was naturally predisposed to create my own underground network through the mountains of my dad's brain and onto North Africa to join the French free forces.

In conclusion, I believe that, with the Holy Spirit's help, we can:

Determine the outcome by choosing our own means of fighting.

From now on, I will refuse to see the outcome of the disease dictated by the means of fighting chosen by the dictatorship.

I stand by my dad with a 'denial of the legitimacy of the dictatorship,' and take a 'posture of noncooperation' toward it.

Determine the outcome by building a democratic space.

From now on, I will find a way to 'progressively grow' an independent society.

I will find the 'democratic space,' where I can have the building blocks for an independent society — outside of the dictator's control.

"How am I going to build this democratic space? With what? Where?" I ask myself.

Kid Marc is comfortable with these questions, so I ask him. "Help me, kid Marc."

"Oh, that's easy," he answers.

"Go on," I say.

"First thing to do is to circumvent his brain."

"Yes, absolutely!" I exclaim. "We have to set up headquarters in a place that's *not* his brain."

"A place outside of the dictatorship's control," says kid Marc.

"Where we can build a democratic space. What else is there that is still living in him that could be a democratic space where we could set up headquarters?" I ask.

"His heart is still beating," says kid Marc.

"That's it! His heart is still alive," I say.

"See, I told you it was easy," says kid Marc with a laugh. "His heart is still alive! It's not that complicated! At least not to me."

"You're a kid," I say laughing. "His heart is still beating. That's huge. That is simple. We have to go for his heart."

"Yeah, I told you."

"How do we get to it?" I ask him.

"Have fun with him. Play with him," is kid Marc's answer.

To a degree he is right. I'm not sure fun and games will be enough to depose the dictator. I know one thing for sure: it is time to go for the heart in every way we can.

"What do you think of when you think of the heart?"

"The land of romance, loyalties and love stories," is kid Marc's answer.

Me: "Yeah! Battles to be fought, damsels to be rescued."

Kid Marc: "Flowers and sunsets."

Me: "The stars."

Kid Marc: "Unending Love."

Me: "Unconditional Love."

Kid Marc: "The love that lays down his life for his brother."

Me: "How do you connect to all that?"

Kid Marc: "Find a secret passage."

Me: "Yeah, the gate to the magic garden."

Kid Marc: "And through the magic forest. Just like the ride d'Artagnan takes in the sequel to *The Three Musketeers* that you are reading."

Me: "What a description that is! That is exactly what we are talking about. Let's read it again."

So I open up the book and read the following passage from *Twenty Years After* by Alexandre Dumas.

"It was a fine spring morning. The birds were singing in the tall trees; the bountiful rays of the sun crossed the forest glades, and looked like curtains of gilded gauze; in other parts, the light scarcely penetrated the thick vault of leaves, and the old oaks, among which the nimble squirrels at the sight of the travelers hurriedly took shelter, were immersed in shade. There arose a perfume from plants, flowers, and leaves, which rejoiced the heart. D'Artagnan wearied with the poisonous air of Paris, said to himself that one ought to be very happy in such a paradise."

Kid Marc: "'Which rejoiced the heart!' I love that. It is so beautiful. Let's find that path to Dad's heart and get him to live out of his heart!"

Me: "OK. We could set up headquarters there and countermand the dictator."

Kid Marc: "And do some damage to his plans and get back the ground."

Me: "High five, man!"

Kid Marc: "Yeah, we'll need courage. What is it that our heroes say on the big screen, or on the pages of our favorite books in the face of insurmountable odds?"

Me: "Take heart."

Kid Marc: "Have courage."

Me: "Just believe."

Kid Marc: "Trust."

Me: "The heart has the power to go where the brain cannot."

Kid Marc: "Because it's smart?"

Me: "No. Because it can love."

Kid Marc: "The heart can love. Reach the love in the heart and the heart will reach out in love."

Kid Marc did not read that somewhere else, in fact, it just bubbles out of him.

I sum up our six-month journey with that phrase: *Reach the love in the heart and the heart will reach back in love.*

That's what kid Marc is trying to tell me.

It is then that I think of a Scripture that I look up in my Bible. It reads as follows:

> *Then Jesus was filled with the joy of the Holy Spirit and said, "I praise you, O Father, Lord of heaven and earth, for hiding these things from the intellectuals and worldly wise and for revealing them to those who are as trusting as little children. Yes, thank you, Father for that is the way you wanted it."*

(Luke 10:21 TLB)

MY HEADQUARTERS
IN THE BATHROOM

I need a way to reach the heart of my dad so he can connect to me, to God, to my mom. And so that he can connect to a part of himself that will make him feel energized to live life — at least for that moment of breakthrough, which sets a precedent for more breakthroughs to happen.

I need an angle to connect with my dad. I need a place that will be our own private space where I can get next to him. Physically, interactively and hands on.

It happens naturally. No deep soul searching here.

Just my father's personal needs.

This is how the bathroom becomes my new headquarters.

My father has very bristly facial growth. During these past weeks and past few years, my mother would use shaving cream and a razor to keep it under control. In the end, this was not that effective and difficult to do. So, I go and buy a good-looking Remington electric shaver with three movable machine heads. Thus begins a daily routine of leading my dad into the bathroom after breakfast.

The sink in the bathroom is decorated with a beautiful painting of flowers that inspires me, and I think inspires all who use the sink. It isn't always easy to 'get' my father into the bathroom, but I do it faithfully.

Sometimes Dad is stuck in his chair at the dining room table and refuses to budge. I am tempted at this point to do something else that is easier and more appealing.

He sits like he is glued to his chair at the dining room table. As I am standing by him, trying to get him up, I feel like I am going against the flow, which makes it harder. But I know that the longer I wait, the more he will sink into his chair.

I loved physics in school, and this situation confirms one of Newton's laws of physics: "An object at rest tends to stay at rest." Which makes it worse.

But, I have made up my mind and it is worth the effort to keep pressing him to stand up and come with me into the bathroom.

My continuous efforts to get him standing can take twenty minutes, so it really comes as a relief once Dad is inside my new headquarters. I can shut the door, and he usually doesn't need to go to the bathroom, so that makes it easier.

"Dad, it's time to shave now. I am going to get this bristly stuff off your face, so stand here."

I have him stand in front of the toilet facing me so I can access both sides of his face. I start off by taking a washcloth and getting it soaked with hot water. I soften his skin a little, leaving the washcloth on his face for a minute. Then I dry up his cheeks and his neck and his lips.

It's just the two of us; I can look into his eyes. He seems to be surrendering to and enjoying this absolute attention. Yes, there are days when he's rambling, but I try to calm him down. "Relax Dad. Just relax. Okay, here we go!"

I reach back to the electric shaver that I have been charging, and turn it on. When the noise of the shaver starts up, lo and behold, I have his attention!

My father can't do much but be present to me. The feel of the shaver on his face is intense, and demanding his full attention. Bzzz..bzzzz. I cannot drift from being present to him for a second.

Come on, I say to myself, *let's get in there!* The passage between his nose and upper lip is always the most demanding to make. The Panama Canal of his face. My father has the toughest, hardest to shave bristles ever, which means that he has to let me mush his face around, over his chin and under his nose. I am awakening his senses and making him feel good.

Of course, I am having fun with this as well, pretending to be flying some kind of airplane over his face, following kid Marc's advice to play with him.

"Brm...brRRm...brmmmmm...brRrmm...bRrm!"

All of this is the set design, the welcoming center to reach the love in his heart. My passion, comes forth very quickly and easily, to talk about how much God loves him and wants to heal him. I want him to know he can trust in the Lord — in spite of this sickness.

Every day, I repeat the same words of life to him:

"Dad, you know Jesus will never leave you nor forsake you. (Hebrews 13:5 NKJ). You are His beloved son, Dad, with whom He is well pleased. (Luke 3:22 NKJ).

"He says, 'Fear not, for I am with you.' (Isaiah 43:5 NKJ). If God is for you, Dad, who can be against you? (Romans 8:31 NKJ).

"You are in the Father's hand and He is greater than all; and no one is able to snatch you out of the Father's hand. (John 10:29 NKJ). He will never leave you, nor forsake you.

"Jesus is bigger than the sickness, and He has got you, Dad. Nothing can separate you from the love of God. Nothing in all creation, and certainly not this sickness, has the power to separate you from His love, Dad." (Romans 8:35-39 NKJ).

I speak confidently, with energy, at a volume that is loud and clear enough to overpower the sound of the shaver. The scriptures are intense and I have to concentrate, look into my father's eyes and mean what I say.

It takes me one minute to declare God's Word to my father. We are very close to each other and always aware of the swaying motion and the motor sound of this fabulous Remington electric shaver.

In fact, to do a good job I am right on top of my dad's face! I want him in a close enough position to receive his true identity as a child of God.

I want God's words to be very personal to him and hope that the pleasurable feelings of being shaved will be a good association with Jesus' words for him.

Not so much to heal his brain.

That's what got him in trouble to start with. Always living out of his intelligence to the detriment of his heart.

It is time to awaken his heart.

"I will awaken the dawn," says the watchman in the Psalms. (Psalm 108:2 NKJ). This is my big plan to reach my father through his senses to his heart.

After all my talks with kid Marc about overcoming dictatorships, the main questions now are:

1. Can the heart set up headquarters and rule from there? *In spite of his brain not working right?*
2. Can his heart be the independent state? *Effectively taking away the ability of the dictator to act?*

If he can live out of his heart, there is life there, a source of life there that can steer him rightly — in spite of his brain not working right. This is my new direction during these past weeks, after trying "to heal his brain."

I've been saying to him over and over, "Remember Dad! Don't listen to the sickness! You don't need to do what the sickness tells you to do."

I am speaking with authority, in the same way as I have spoken with the animals and the children, back in Tulsa, believing they understand and hear me perfectly clearly.

"Dad, you are a child of God. You are following Jesus and doing what you would normally do."

"BrRRm...bRrm!" The shaver is going in the background.

"You just tell the sickness: 'No I am not following you! I am healed. In Jesus name be gone! I am trusting in the Lord with all my heart, and not leaning on this sickness or on my own understanding."

I am using a verse that can be the springboard for my new direction. It is the mother lode of wisdom for my father. He knows this verse well, very well, and I am totally counting on him knowing it by 'heart' to succeed. It is a scripture that Dad has memorized.

"Trust in the Lord with all your heart, and lean not on your own understanding." (Proverbs 3:5 NKJ)

It is a scripture that Dad often quoted to me years ago, along with the rest of the passage: "In all your ways acknowledge Him and He shall direct your paths. Do not be wise in your own eyes; fear the Lord and depart from evil. It will be health to your flesh, and strength to your bones." (Proverbs 3:6-8 NKJ)

"Trust in the Lord," I start by saying as a primer for my dad to jump in and sure enough he echoes back, "with all your heart, and lean not on your own understanding!"

We say it together, and then we say the whole verse again. Together. "Trust in the Lord with all your heart, and lean not on your own understanding!"

When this happens, I want to jump up and down from the sheer excitement of our success. But, I stay on a steady keel, as we stand there in the refreshed bathroom air. Caution dictates, as I would probably knock my dad over or freak him out.

Three weeks after establishing our new routine I see a gleam in my dad's eyes.

"Thank you, Marc for taking good care of me," is what he says.

I am blown away, and totally surprised. His comment is clearly spoken from somewhere not under the sickness's control. My father is filled with gratitude.

"I love you, Dad," is what I tell him, still blown away and humbled.

My father looks at me happily, and we pause here, with God's kindness wrapped around us in this sweet moment.

Yes, kid Marc is here too, smiling about the great connection between the two of us.

Reach the love in the heart and the heart will reach back in love. That's what kid Marc is trying to tell me.

JANUARY

There are more victories, but they don't take place without going through several challenges during January, in the new year of 2013.

Everything becomes harder in January — harder to let go of promoting my book; harder to sleep in a twin bed with my feet sticking out the foot of the bed; harder to live surrounded by these clothes that belong to my mother and father that they surely will not wear again; and harder to breathe in a room used for the storage of my parents' extras from a bygone era.

"Me being here is a gift from God you know," I say when my mother seems more preoccupied with her stuff than about me.

There is a large artist's rendering on the wall, right beside my bed. It is of a one-man sailboat being tossed and turned in the raging ocean waves, buckling down in a fierce wind. The sailboat is moving through these distressing conditions with a beaten down gib, no other sails, no human in sight, cold salt water splashing everywhere. No sun, gray sky. Not even someone on deck braving the weather.

I'm getting tired of seeing this picture day after day in my room. It's wearing me down. I need some relief.

"Mom, I am really tired of seeing this picture in my room. May I take it down?"

"Well, this is a picture of Chichester passing Cape Horn, which has its home here in our computer room."

What happened after that, I would learn, was a reaction in my mother resulting from the long-term contact with my father's sickness. This is a need in my mom to hang on to what she has.

But for my part, I need my own space where I can center myself again. Now that my humble and much smaller (than I am used to) space is being unexpectedly threatened, it produces an argument in me. My mom tells me how very grateful she is that I agreed to come and live there, and help her with Dad. So how come all this stuff in the room is suddenly more important than me?

All I am asking is about the picture! Now, I have to defend 'my room' which is basically all I have left in the world, after leaving everything behind, coming here to Florida to live in my parents' apartment.

Did I argue about the picture? No! We got past the picture real fast. At this point, I am ready to duke it out.

"What do you mean, computer room? This *is* my room. I'm here to help you and Dad. I gave up my house, my friends and now I have to fit in here with all your clothes in the closet, in the drawers, your books on the shelves and sleep on this narrow twin-size bed. Me being here is a gift from God you know."

I topped off the pleading of my case: "Mom, you have to at least appreciate where I'm coming from!"

But the problem is not solved with my mother using this sort of logic. The "put yourself in my moccasins" approach doesn't go very far. At first, I think: "Maybe it's because I'm not *wearing* moccasins!" I look down at the slippers my mother insists that I wear in the house, to protect the carpet, then shake my head. *No, that isn't it.*

My mom has told me many times about her beloved Père — Father — and his reaction to the questioning of his authority: "Ne me contredit pas." "Don't contradict me," was his answer to all who challenged his authority. "*Don't* contradict me."

He had a strong will; he was a hero of the French Resistance; a recipient of the Legion d'Honneur. His unbending resolve enabled him to accomplish great feats of courage, especially since he had to have his left arm amputated during World War I.

This character trait, inherited from her father, was for my mother the only rule of engagement during difficult times. Her strong will unfortunately also exhibits a stubborn attitude, to the detriment of her health. My mother's primary care doctor is recommending a colonoscopy, but my mom does not want to take more tests. I am continuing to pray for her healing, of course, but remain ambivalent about her attitude toward her doctor.

I know that we will have to be of one mind and spirit to pull off taking care of Dad and helping him get beyond the hold of the Alzheimer's. But my requests for a relationship based on mutual respect are having trouble being welcomed, accepted, received, and decoded.

TEAM BUILDING

I assume my mom will be eager to join in my plans — given my experience in the business world for 25 years and in leadership for 4 years with Toastmasters' International.

In our Club in Tulsa — THE POETS, an acronym for *The Pursuers of Excellence Toastmasters* — I did research and gave a speech for a 'training presentation' on Team Building.

I found four essential components needed to support a team. We base our leadership style on:

THE SERVANT-LEADERSHIP MODEL FOR TEAM BUILDING

1. **Continuous communication among Team members** *while searching for answers.*
2. **Consistent availability and willingness** *to be counted on.*
3. **Commitment to the priorities** *of the Team's goals.*
4. **Personal interaction based on** *a mutual relationship of accountability.*

Combined, these four essential elements create 'servant-leadership,' which is leadership designed to lead — by edifying others, by building people up, by setting them free and by giving them wings to fly.

No one person is dominating and team relationships are mutual, not 'big person — little person.'

So I am thinking, *having mutual relationship is one of the essential building blocks of teamwork*, while my mom, in turn, is thinking: *Don't contradict me.*

Two kinds of leadership style in a room that is too small for both of them.

"This town is too small for both of us," as they say in Westerns.

I think since it is my room, my point of view can rule in this situation.

Turns out, these two twin beds have a much-valued history to my mother. These are the same beds from our apartment in Paris, on which I had slept when I was younger, much younger, like eight, nine and 10 and up into my 20s — after that they were moved to Connecticut and later to Michigan.

The last time I slept on one of these beds was back in 1983. Regardless of the 30-year stretch, for my mother the word "beds" triggers off a speech as essential to one's cherished values as the Proclamation of Independence was to our ancestors.

"These are fine beds! Everyone who sleeps here always has such a good night's sleep. You should be very happy."

These conversations, I am sad to say, are repeated on several occasions.

My dad is wandering around in his own world and my mom is valuing the beds more than the fact that I'm actually here in person to help.

This is, I guess, also the reason why I am here. Things have gotten out of hand for my mom and dad.

I wonder if I can find out how things got out of hand from my father's journals on the book shelves. Most of the 5 to 6 composition notebooks he has written are in his small handwriting, in pencil, and are most difficult to read. The few passages I discover that I can understand talk about past situations in which my father addresses the validity of his decisions. He raises concerns and is writing to find answers to his questions.

Here on these shelves are also the many books and study guides that inspired my father's faith, and index cards of Scriptures he has written.

I pray that I will find inspiration for myself as I peruse these books. Brennan Manning, Brother Andrew, and Mother Theresa inspire me to press on. Sometimes it feels as if they are actually present and cheering me on.

With my father and mother's relationship shifting as it has been, my mom is holding on, as strongly as she can, to how they had lived their lives together in this house since 1990. She is holding on to their routines, their connections, and their identity. This room represents the life they share.

The picture, I found out later, has a special significance for my mother. I thought it represented their great adventures at sea when they lived on their own sailboat for 13 months. That was the best time in my mom's whole life, she has always told me.

In point of truth, when my father was first setting up his office in his new Paris location, my mother chose this print, had it framed, and offered it to him for the wall facing his desk.

"He was very happy with it. It really meant a lot to him. As for sailing around the world on my own, that's something I would never want to do. I would not want to go out on my own for one day!"

(This information is revealed to me by my mother on a casual afternoon in June of 2015, two years after my father's death. Light years in the future from my 2013 present reality.)

I think this picture of the boat holding on in the storm is an image my mom has related to for the last three years, during which she has had to keep a steadfast eye and a constant watch on my father.

Unfortunately for me and my mom, the picture has come to represent a state of frustration, "For crying out loud," as they say.

While everything hasn't been a bed of roses with my father, I do feel a sense of love for him and I have compassion for him.

But I do not have my mother's feelings for my father. All of a sudden I am getting tired and worn out, and I need an environment that will reflect my needs.

In Tulsa, I had been sleeping on my son Josh's, $800 queen-size bed with his 800 count Egyptian cotton sheets, that he was able to pay for thanks to a $10,000 gift he received from his beloved Grandma Corrine after her husband died.

I spent 32 months sitting at his desk writing *The Coolness of Josh* on his laptop. I had a large home with a half-acre backyard, surrounded by beautiful giant pecan trees.

I made friends with the squirrels who raced each other up and down the bark of the giant trees, jumping from one branch to another, at the most perilous heights. I was surrounded by the song of birds and the presence of rabbits, which would come right up to me on my front lawn.

In the back yard, surrounded by a circle of fresh pine trees, sat a magnificent Hot Springs hot tub, crowned by roses growing beside it. Sitting with the jets on, feeling the massage of the bubbles, I delighted in the surrounding visual feast and the fragrant smell of the red and orange roses.

Topping off such a friendly environment all around me, of beauty and peace, I had the wonderful presence of my beloved son Josh, still in the house with me. I had made a giant 24" x 36" poster photo of him, smiling and happy, which sat in my den. How many times I talked to him, about the funny stuff and heavy stuff going on in my life, the same things we used to talk about all the time.

Now, the picture I'm looking at is not of my smiling, happy Josh, which is still in Tulsa, but of a stormy sea, with Chichester's boat chugging along under an ominous churning sky, without him even being on deck!

I cannot relate to this picture. It represents isolation and loneliness.

What am I going to do, have compassion for him?

Start a *conversation* with him?

"Hey, Chester! Hello! Can you hear me, Chester?"

No reply.

Why am I not surprised? I shout louder over the wind and the waves: "Hey man! Need anything?!"

I think I actually hear him say, "About now I need some lovin'!"

To which I answer, "I hear you, my friend. Just stay alive!"

He needs a big hug, but how to get it to him? Only God can do that, and now I am in the same boat — no pun intended.

Maybe, on a deeper level, the invisible man in the boat is my father, grasping for strength and meaning in the vortex of a powerful drain.

My father loved to sail.

We rented a sailboat several times.

When the wind is right and the sails are tight, the boat, leaning over, cuts into the water in a straight line. But in the storm, the waves rise and lift the boat up high, so you are looking down into a great dark hollow and then they dip, and from the deck you go down and are looking up at this 20-foot wave above you, that is in the next second, going to be lifting you back up 20 feet.

The sails get twisted and agitated, shaken spasmodically, unwrapped and over wrapped. Unpurposed. Undone. Because the wind doesn't work the same and the boat isn't working the same.

What a perilous, useless feeling, trying to find a steady course at the top of each wave. The water splashing on our heads is the only thing that is steady as we drop down again. As long as we make it back up to the top of that wave, we are still alive.

In the Aegean Sea, the Swift family almost had a shipwreck, on the sailboat my father had rented. It demanded our complete attention, to stay balanced, to brace for the waves.

We made it. A man on land saw our flare, went to ask a fishing boat for help; they came out, sent a rope and hauled us back to port. The boat didn't sink, we didn't drown.

So that is now my goal with my dad — to make it into port okay. I want none of this going down in the ocean stuff, no reports of being lost at sea. No, we are going to get this battered vessel home safe into the harbor.

Overcoming the forces of nature can be an exciting challenge and very fulfilling for a man or a woman. But overcoming the forces of evil requires the accompaniment of a greater power. The accompaniment of the Lord Jesus: "Then He arose and rebuked the wind and the raging of the water. And they ceased, and there was a calm. But He said to them, 'Where is your faith?' And they were afraid and marveled, saying to one another, 'Who can this be? For He commands even the winds and water, and they obey Him!'" (Luke 8:24-25 NKJ).

The one who created everything is Lord over all his creation — even the part that went wrong because man handed over his authority to the serpent-devil.

"By him all things were made and without him, nothing was made that was made." Jesus, the Son of the Father who brought us all back to the Father's love.

Yes, more than ever I need the accompaniment of Jesus. I also need an environment of love, where I can receive an 'epipipto' — what is called in Greek — a love hug from the Holy Spirit. And I probably I need some compassion and a hug from my mom too.

TRUST

What can I do to keep my sanity? Of course, I pray and I journal. Most of all, I wish for a friend to talk with.

I call my cousin Elise in France. We have developed a close relationship over the years, which has continued to this day. After my dad had died, she came from France and was very helpful. But for now, she has heard about my mission to help my dad, and says:

"It's very beautiful the work you are doing with your father. Uncle Bob and 'Auntie' Monique have always been the best part of our lives. You represent all of us with your love for uncle Bob."

She is very encouraging. I share with her my frustration about the living arrangements. My cousin's advice is: "Just get your own stuff moved from Tulsa as soon as possible. Move out the old beds, move in your bed. You need your own desk! You can't live like that!"

While it is great talking with her, putting her advice into action is easier said than done.

The issue goes deeper than a matter of the arrangements in the room. My heart is crying out for a Mom with a caring heart. These confrontations set off a quiet phone call at night or early the next morning to my friend Mary in Tulsa, who had already lived the nightmare with her own mother.

Mary had actually ended up moving out of her house into her mother's house to take care of her for six years. The 'six years' part seems completely out of the ballpark to me. I have been living with my parents for six weeks and I am already going ballistic.

"I have to wipe up my father's poop, take off his Depends underwear, put them in a baggie, put on a new Depends, get him to let me pull up his pants again, all the while being obliged to view my father's private parts over and over."

Mary understands my dismay.

"I felt the same frustration," she says. "It is such a sickening task, and it is without reward or appreciation. I was alone, but your mom is there. She has to really appreciate you being there."

"It's a mixed bag. I do really know that my mom is grateful for me being here. But there is also this attitude where she just says to me: 'I've been doing it for the past three years.'"

"Right!" Mary says with a chuckle.

"My answer to that is: 'He's your husband. That's what a wife does. She takes care of her husband! Bob is not my husband.' To which she says: 'Any good son would do the same thing.'"

"Marc, you are a good son. Look at how you loved Josh, and guided him to being happy and full of joy again! And you are a great Dad! So, yeah, you are a good son. Didn't you tell me you had a brother? If any good son would do the same thing, then how does she feel about him not doing the same thing? Why isn't he there? Isn't he just as much a good son? Couldn't your mother have paid for his expenses? Each day it is your choice to give or not to give. Your father wouldn't feel that you are under any obligation to do this. So to feel like it's an obligation or duty...It is not."

"That's the thing." I say about the good son thing: "How about the good dad thing? He was never there for me. In fact, he insulted me, he said I was a screw-up and I'd never amount to much. And now I'm in the bathroom wiping up his..."

"I am really with you Marc. I really understand your frustration. I went through the same ordeal with my mother. I had no life of my own. She just became more and more demanding. Before I knew it, I was stuck, and it took a lot of work to set some boundaries and find a way to rise above it."

"Thanks Mary. I do feel stuck. I threw up the other night. I wrenched my guts out. What kind of boot camp training is this? I've never been in anything this hard. It never lets up."

"It sounds like you signed up for much more than you realized. No one should have to see his father's nudity. At your age especially, to have to take care of your father's hygiene? It should be a time of honor between the two of you. A time when he blesses you because he's proud of you."

"Yeah, that was the idea. The problem was that all our lives were so messed up. That's why I wanted to find pathways of healing for him. Remember the movie I showed to our Toastmasters club in Tulsa? I talked about the power of personal presence. This is personal presence on steroids! I came in saying, 'Okay, I'll stay.' Now I'm feeling more like the guy in the marketplace at the beginning of Disney's Aladdin movie — you know, who says, 'come closer,' and then the camera presses right up against his *nose* and he shouts, 'Too close! Too close!!'"

Mary laughs. I laugh, and we have a good laugh together. It feels great.

Time to get off the phone and Mary has some parting words. "After Josh's death, it worked because you loved him. There you are alone again in a sense, acting by your faith, with your sights on healing your father. You are very brave, yet what a trial of your self-esteem and well-being."

We talk more for several evenings in a similar way. Talking with Mary always helps me get back on track, and things do get better. The grace of God has a huge amount to do with this change.

It's funny because back in our Toastmasters' Club in Tulsa, I had been able to encourage Mary and help her believe that God would help her get out of a seemingly impossible financial dead end. I prayed with her that healing prayer that I just really believe in.

Praying for healing is a lifestyle to me. My only prerequisite is that I need to feel some kind of love or compassion for that person.

There is a good ending to this story. She got out of her financial trouble amazingly well. Now Mary is helping me because she had been through the same experience with her mother. Cool how the right people come around to help you when you really need them.

FINDING MY BALANCE

One thing my mom has said to me: "Of course, you won't have to worry about the finances. I will take care of everything you need." Undoubtedly, this made it possible for me to be there, but it gave rise to a question in my mind. Was I now putting up with the current 'inconveniences' as a sort of trade-off?

Actually, I never see it that way. I am not here to compromise or to prove something. Psalm 127 says: "Unless the Lord builds the house, they labor in vain who build it. Unless the Lord guards the city, the watchman stays awake in vain." (NKJ). I am trusting God to build the house, and that will only happen when I am true to the Marc He created me to be. I need to be myself in order to reach my dad and find pathways of healing for him.

I am also taking my mom literally about the money. Being able to communicate with my mom is an expression of my needs that I figure will soon get resolved.

My weapons of choice have always been to write, so I write out a two-part script of what I would like to *have happen* with my mother.

Mom: *"Hey Marc!"*
Me: *"Hey Mom!"*
Mom: *"Dad and I are so happy that you're here."*
Me: *(This is true, I knew this. My mother had told me this.)*
Mom: *"I am proud of all you've done and now that you are here to help us, I am very grateful. I was always so proud of Dad that*

I never wanted you to see him like this. It is a difficult thing to clean cars as you have done in your business, looking at dirt all day long. I feel like you are doing the same thing here, only worse! I am sorry to ask you to clean him up, to wipe his poop and see him naked. That really is my responsibility, but I just can't do it, I am too tired.

"Can you help me please? I want you to see Dad in an honorable way, rather than in what could feel shameful to you. What you are doing with Dad is very appreciated, to be available 24 hours a day like this. I am so grateful you are here. The Lord bless you as you undertake your new mission with Dad."

Me: *"Amen. May the Lord bless you, Mom."*

That is my script, and writing it helps me believe a dialog like this can actually happen.

Back to my script of hopes and needs for my room.

Mom: *"Please make yourself at home, Marc. You just move out my clothes and Dad's clothes on that first rack in the closet and the clothes in the dresser so you can have more room. In fact, you will be doing me a favor. I've been meaning to give away those clothes for ages!"*

Me: *"All right! I can even drop those clothes off for you later if that will help."*

Mom: *"Thank you."*

Upon contemplating my script, I think, *This would be a great start!*

Next, I need to reaffirm my friendship with my true father in the faith, Dr. T.L. Osborn. I send him a copy of my book *The Coolness of Josh.* On February 8, 2013, I get a letter back from him thanking me for my gift:

Dear Brother Marc:

"It is God Himself who has made us what we are and given us new lives from Jesus Christ; and long ages ago he planned that we should spend these lives in helping others." Ephesians 2:10, The Living Bible.

On behalf of Dr. T. L. and Dr. LaDonna Osborn, thank you for the personally autographed gift copy of your book *The Coolness of Josh*. The Osborns sincerely appreciate your thoughtfulness and sharing with them this beautiful and heart moving story about your precious son, Josh.

No life is without purpose. Josh's life certainly had great purpose! We are sure that your story of Josh's extraordinary life will relate to many people and help them to more clearly understand God's deep Love for us all.

May God bless you, brother Marc, as you continue to minister His love to people.

Sincerely in Christ,

Pat Lovern,
Executive Assistant to Dr. T.L. Osborn
OSBORN Ministries International

The amazing thing to me is that I receive the letter on February 12 and two days later, on February 14, I receive an email saying Dr. Osborn died in his sleep. I feel that he waited to receive my book before dying.

This letter is a great honor. If I had waited one more week, I would have missed him. But I didn't. He received it and he made sure to send me a letter with his blessing in return, a week before he went to be with his Father God.

I turn to a book written by my spiritual father, Dr. T.L. Osborn, called *Healing the Sick*. He reaffirmed that God means what He says, that sickness comes from the devil, but that the devil is defeated and that I have been given authority over Satan.

"They overcame him by the blood of the Lamb and by the word of their testimony." (Revelation 12: 11 NKJ). My French translation says: "By the truth of their testimony." The truth of our testimony is the legitimacy of God's truth and the illegitimacy of Satan's lies, which he disguises as our own thoughts to make us think his thoughts are *our* ideas. As soon as we agree with him and believe him, we are rendering void the legitimacy of what God has said, "So shall My word be that goes forth from My mouth: it shall not return to Me void, but it shall accomplish what I please, and it shall prosper in the thing for which I sent it." (Isaiah 55:11 NKJ)

The way you overcome Satan is to confront all doubts and human reasoning — such as, that it is God's will for you to suffer or that it is not God's will to heal everybody — and say as Jesus did, "It is written." (Luke 4:4 NKJ).

T.L. Osborn says: "Say what God says. Satan can never endure that. He is a defeated foe, and he knows it. He has known it ever since Jesus rose victorious over death and hell. He has always sought to prevent the church from making this discovery. Satan has always had to obey the command of believers who use God's word against him. When he finds that we have discovered the secret of using 'It is written,' his surrender is certain. All evil spirits have to leave by the same Word. Then add Isaiah 53:4-5: 'By his stripes, I am healed; He has borne my sicknesses and carried my diseases. The chastisement needful to obtain peace and well-being for me is upon him.'" (Osborn, T.L. *Healing the Sick*. Tulsa: Harrison House, 1992.)

The truth is that I need this boost to be strong in my spirit, in order to win the battle which is about to begin. I have months ahead of directly confronting evil which impacts me considerably. Physically it is the hardest thing I've ever had to do.

THE MARX BROTHERS JOIN US

The humbling task of having to take care of my own father's personal hygiene two to three times a day is way beyond the boundaries of anything I ever thought I would have to do. Every day I am in the bathroom waiting on him; often at times I definitely do not want to be there, waiting to see if I need to clean up and change his underwear (code for Depends). I use baby wipes and even with them the job is difficult. But I think you get the picture.

I had two sons and I changed their diapers many times. They wiggled and squirmed; it was sometimes a challenge. But it was still baby stuff next to this.

Instead of cooperating with me by standing still, letting me finish what I am doing, my father starts acting deliberately contrary to me. Right in the middle of the baby wipe moment, he starts turning his body sideways and lifts his leg up and puts it over into the bathtub. Worse even than this — because he is at least still standing — in the middle of my baby wipe moment, he decides to sit back down on the toilet seat, or determine that now is the time to reach down and pull up his pants.

These confrontations with his determined contrariness, defiance, and mockery become a habitual routine. The only antics like this that I have experienced in any form are in movies with the Marx Brothers. Coincidentally the Marx Brothers played an influential part in my childhood. At the age of nine, while living in Paris, my mother took me to see *Monkey Business*, *Duck Soup* and

A Day at the Races. I grew up laughing at their zaniness, and seeing all thirteen of their movies.

Groucho was the more intellectual one, looking a little ridiculous in his loose suit, striding forward with every step looking like his legs were trying to catch up with his chest, grinning, with a painted-on mustache and eyebrows.

Chico was more dimensional and likable, with his high energy mischievous wit and charm, loving to pun, speaking English with a revved-up Italian accent, wearing a leprechaun's hat and a jacket too small to fit him.

Harpo's appearance was most striking, looking like a street urchin, with a mop of curly hair and ragged clothes. He showed up often wearing a big overcoat, out of which he produced oversize objects such as a blow torch, or big scissors. And to top it all off, he did not speak. He expressed himself with faces and whistles and gestures, often losing patience and causing havoc.

Mixed together, the brothers were high powered chaos-driven mischief, which is just what I am experiencing with my dad and which makes me think of them. As things begin daily to spiral out of control, it seems like the Marx Brothers become more and more interested in joining us, which for a while, they do. My father's daily run-arounds become an irresistible invitation for them to join the party.

Harpo was bald, but on camera, he wore a bright carrot colored, curly-haired wig. When he wasn't acting, he could take it off and have a normal life because no one recognized him. Well, this is definitely not *normal*. The Marx brothers aren't making me laugh anymore, like they used to, even though I was a big fan when I was younger.

My father, and consequently, me, become the center of their chaos driven run-around, here, in the bathroom.

"Who me?" and "What?! This isn't the way you do it?" are my father's standard responses to whatever I say.

"Dad we are going to brush your teeth now," I say actually holding his hand while helping him to hold his toothbrush. "Now you put it in your mouth, like this," I say, letting go of my hold.

Instead of the anticipated action of him brushing his teeth, he talks. He stops, and looks at me and says, "What?! This isn't the way you do it!?"

My father is now using his toothbrush to clean out the soap dish while holding the soap bar in his other hand, and using his mouth to back it up. "This isn't the way you do it?"

These are the comments my father is making, as he is doing the opposite of what I want him to do. St. Francis would be considering anger management seminars had he been present.

"Don't listen to the sickness," I tell him. "Dad, you have to do what you normally do. Ok, don't you put the toothbrush in your mouth to brush your teeth?"

My patience is strained.

"Let me show you," I say, taking the toothbrush, rinsing out the soap from it, putting back the soap dish, and the bar of soap from his hand, getting soap all over my fingers which I now have to rinse, then trying again with the toothbrush.

"Okay, Dad, we are brushing your teeth. Hold the brush like this. Wait, the toothpaste washed off, I have to put more on. The toothpaste has to go on the brush, Dad. You just put your brush back in the mug? Dad, don't pick up the soap again. What are you turning on the water for? Now you're washing the soap?"

My nerves are sizzling like eggs cracked open on the burning hot cement of a New York sidewalk during the most unbearable day of summer. My patience is burned up and my short fuse is down to a smoldering taper, in the midst of this sweltering insanity and chaos. This is anger-inducing behavior to even the gentlest soul.

Just when I think I can take no more, we have company. That is to say, I have the privilege of an uninvited special appearance by Groucho Marx, and his sidekick, Chico and *his* sidekick, Harpo.

Now there are five of us in this little room, barely wide enough for two.

"Come and gett'a your tickets! Surprise'a performance just'a today!" I recognize Chico's voice and his trademark Italian accent.

"The Marx Brothers! Now making a special appearance titled, 'In the Bathroom.' In living color, and in 3-D."

Groucho is right there with us, holding up his token cigar, telling me to "get a real job," and prompting my father to "be a man and pull up your pants!"

Then he chants, "Whatever it is, I'm against it! I'm ahhh-gainst it!"

Looking over his shoulder at my father, Groucho adds another side crack: "You don't have to put up with this, you know! You should think about your reputation."

Meanwhile, Chico is setting up shop in the bathtub. He successfully convinces my father that he is better off cleaning up in the bathtub, saying with his Italian accent: "Come on'a boss, it's a shower time. Stepp'a right in." Chico shows him how to get his leg in the bathtub, and my father is naturally eager to comply.

"That's a champ. We clean'a you up real good. You'll see! Get your tootsie, fruitsie!"

As I struggle to get my dad's leg back out of the tub, Harpo is holding his nose, unrolling the toilet paper, squinting his eyes and, turning on the faucets in the sink, flicking on and off the lights, and turning on the fan. Then he stashes the toothbrushes and the mug holder inside his overcoat.

I am humiliated in this situation, as my father is running around in opposites to my directions, and making a mockery out of my well-intentioned efforts to take care of him.

Whatever virtue is in my humble service is being defaced by the temptation to be angry, or to be impatient, or the temptation to inter-space my kind words with negative, derogatory ones and to raise my voice. Here we go with the frustration and anger management issues again.

I can only handle so much, and this feels like more than I can bear.

Time to throw in the towel.

Wait a minute! What is Harpo doing right now?

He is throwing *all* the towels over to Chico in the shower.

"Ha-ha-ha," Chico bursts out laughing and adds, "That'sa what I call a good'a catch!"

Groucho turns to me and says: "You don't need this! You should move to Florida and get out of this business. There's plenty of pretty girls down there, you know."

Somehow the talk of pretty girls sets Harpo and Chico in motion and they run out of the bathroom, leaving the door ajar. Groucho turns in the doorway for one last remark and says, raising his eyebrows: "I have *my* reputation to think about," and then he leaves in a huff.

We are left alone to make our way out of the bathroom.

Unbelievably, standing in the hallway, on the blue and white striped carpet, the still monotony is too much of a contrast and not the relief I hoped for. The madness — now being denied altogether by my father, who is standing there with his classic 'who me?' look on his face — is never addressed.

My mother will never believe me. Groucho was not even smoking. So there is no cigar smoke in the air to prove they were here.

No, I will have to say something along these lines: "It was like The Marx Brothers were right there with us in the bathroom!" I will have to use the 'like' word. This completely discredits what actually happened — although it might lead to a fun discussion about her taking me to see *Monkey Business* when I was nine.

My singular morning encounters with the Marx Brothers are repeated on several occasions. Each time, there is never quite enough evidence to prove to my mother that they have actually been here, and my father isn't telling.

When it comes to the shower in the bathroom though, Chico did make a positive impression, as is evidenced one day soon after, when my mother wants my father to take a shower. She asks me to help. So I put on my swimming trunks and climb into the bathtub.

My mom says to me: "Don't you need to be out *here* to help him get in?"

"Just ask him to get in," I answer confidently.

"Bob, can you get into the bathtub?" my mom asks him, a little incredulous.

The moment she finishes speaking, my dad willingly complies. Thanks to Chico, he is well versed at putting his leg over the side of the bathtub.

He is, of course, responding to Chico's voice: "Come on in'na boss. We clean'a you up real good! Get your tootsie-fruitsie!"

My dad and Chico are already good friends by now and so, of course, it is easy, putting his leg over the side of the bathtub.

That famous day, getting my dad into the bathtub is a piece of cake. My mom is delighted. Thank you, Chico.

The shower is going and the water is warm and relaxing. I wash his hair. He washes what he can reach himself, but rinsing the soap out is a little more of a challenge since it is hard to get him to move in a circular motion.

Interestingly, he has his tough-guy attitude on, cleaning himself up and rinsing off like he is offloading bad guys, decisively using his hands to shove off the water from his skin.

So here we are: I am wearing swimming trunks and my dad is naked in the shower yet he's acting like a gritty crime boss in the boardroom, giving orders and moving off the soap suds with finality.

His face is totally serious and he is acting totally stable, not doing anything contrary or giving me a hard time. Is getting in the shower something he has really wanted to do all along? Chico was there calling him in, and now Dad is happy and getting what he wants? He is acting very satisfied. I always did like Chico, and I sure appreciate being able to relax.

The two of us are a riot, me in my hip bathing suit and Dad reenacting some sort of Mr. Big moment. He could have been wearing a tie — it would have been the same. At least he is using the soap for what it is meant for, which lightens my heart. Not sure how I am reaching *his* heart yet, but I enjoy the lift.

We come to the end of our Water World experience and my dad is happy as can be as I turn off the water. My mom is there to greet him as he is now adroitly lifting his leg out of the bathtub, and casually stepping out of the shower and enjoying being wrapped in her big white towel.

"There you go, Bobby! You did that so well!" she says, wrapping him in the big towel.

"You are so sweet!" my father says.

"You are all wet! My bear, let's dry you up!"

"Oh, that's just what a bear needs!" answers my father.

LAUNDRY TIME

I find further relief that afternoon, as it is laundry time. Ah, the laundry room. A place of rest — functional in its ability, yet liberating in its time constraints.

Most people think, "Man, now I have to wait around for the laundry?" Actually here at the Cloisters Condos, people will load up, start up, note the time, leave and come back...or not. Yes, some would forget and hopefully come back later at one point, after I was gone.

Not yours truly. I appreciate this block of time and make it into a sacred space during which I have time for myself.

I can not 'go back' and hang with my parents anyway — there is always something that will come up, I will be delayed coming back, the clothes will be jammed in the washer, so, not an option. I receive this necessary time off with joy.

The whole experience is an outing of sorts. I have to go one floor down with the metal frame basket on wheels that my mother uses for her laundry, with the clothes packed into 1970's nylon Equinox sailing bags, one blue and one yellow. With the cart, I need to take the elevator, but once on the fourth floor, there is an open balcony to traverse as I make my way to the front of the building where the laundry room is located.

Along the way, I walk through a magical, narrow area, where the black iron fence is flanked with two gigantic pots taking up half the hallway and pouring out into an even larger area with the most gorgeous flower shoots of all colors. This is almost a gate with an invitation on it: to knock on the door and visit the undoubtedly enchanting and happy lady within, whose flowers, it seems, love to celebrate life.

I never knock, of course, or run into the mysterious occupant during my travels back and forth, whose flowers I admire. In fact, most of the time, the apartment is dark with no sign of activity. I receive this tenderness nonetheless because it is so lacking in my life.

I set up shop on the wrought-iron bench facing the laundry room door, feeling wrapped up in 'some kind of wonderful' love hug from the Holy Spirit. This bench is in a tucked-away space, on the outdoor balcony, in the shade in the fresh Florida heat which I have come to enjoy more and more.

The palm trees and styled architecture of the area are very inspiring and remind me of my younger days in Europe, and especially in Florence, Italy, with its red-tiled rooftops. "Thank you, Jesus!"

I carry a little notebook which I pull out and in which I write my thoughts about different ideas for maybe writing a book about this journey I am on with my dad.

Most of all, I write down the words that I receive from the Lord in this contemplative hideaway. They are always encouraging and filled with promises for 'a future and a hope' here in Florida, for happiness and prosperity.

Pulling out the clothes from the dryer and folding them in piles is the final panache, before I make my way back, loaded with fresh clothes to the Swift's apartment on the fifth floor.

I return feeling refreshed and renewed. My mother is always so delighted and almost surprised that I know how to fold clothes after doing my own laundry for 25 years. "You do such a good job folding all these clothes! Now Dad has fresh tee-shirts to wear and clean pajamas."

Soon upon arriving I became adamant about dressing my father in proper clothes during the day, and not letting him lounge around in his pajamas. I started a consistent routine of going from the bathroom after 'shaving' into his bedroom, to put on pants with his favorite belt, a button-down shirt, socks, and slippers. I think he enjoys being dressed up, judging by the look on his face when he catches sight of himself in the mirror.

His right eyebrow tilts upwards and his head nods up and down with a satisfied look, 'You are a *good looking* guy.'

My mother enters the room with a gasp of delight, only reinforcing his sentiment, and which gives us a moment of pleasure. "Bobby, don't you look dashing!"

"Dad is one handsome guy," I reply. These are special, and especially short, moments after a fair amount of work has been put toward this end result. These are moments to be cherished.

On several evenings after doing laundry, my mother, feeling more invigorated by the fresh clothes, is talkative. This is how I learn about the event that was such a trauma to my dad that it literally sent him into shock.

STEPS FORWARD

The rain is pouring down and pounding the windows and the roof.

Dad is in bed and Mom and I retreat to the white couch and coffee table in the back of the living room, to sit underneath the big windows that are behind us.

"You know, it's thanks to Dad that we have this roof."

"No, I did not know that," I say with interest.

"He was chairman of the Board, and he insisted on having an appraisal company check the roof after it started leaking in several places. Many people opposed him, saying it would be too expensive, but when the report came in, it was clear that a new roof would have to be installed. So it is thanks to him that we have this roof."

"That was a good achievement. With this kind of rain, you need a strong roof."

"Getting the new roof built was a huge success for him as chairman of the Board. But as time went on, the board members changed and forgot what he had done. He had some people against him, who wanted to do things their way."

"Board members against him?" I say.

"One night after a Board meeting, he came home so pale. A group of them had ganged up on him and asked him to step down, right in front of the whole board. I wasn't there that night; I had a really bad cold. It seems that no one stood up to defend him or to moderate the proceedings."

"What a shock!"

"It was such a shock to him. Everyone thought he was such a gentleman, he had such good manners, and you know how Dad was very respectful and kind. This mutiny just came out of nowhere and threw him for a loop."

"Had he started showing signs of memory loss or acting less competent? Was that what they were picking up on?" I asked.

"Maybe, but he was so used to being well treated by everybody." So was Mom. In a conversation with Debbie, the property manager, about my dad, she said that at the last meeting, she had "straightened out the residents who attacked your dad." She loved my mom and would say to me: "When I grow up, I want to be just like your mom."

"Dad was all pale? If he was used to you being there, that must have been difficult for him to handle. Being all alone."

"I know. I wish I had been there. I hate the devil. He took advantage of me not feeling well to hurt Dad."

"It sucks. I bet this is the trauma that set the Alzheimer's in motion. The devil's dictatorship wants to take Dad down, but we are not going to let that happen. The Book of Revelation says, 'The accuser of our brethren has been cast down. They overcame him by the blood of the Lamb and by the word of their testimony.' (Revelation 12:11 NKJ). Jesus has already defeated him. We are going to find a way to help Dad."

"You really think so?" she says.

"Well, you are into healing. You were part of Charles and Frances Hunter's healing ministry. What was it they always said? "If one method of prayer or healing doesn't work, try another one. Don't give up until you find one that does work. There is always a way! Nothing is impossible with God."

"That's right, they trained us. We were both healing ministers during their rallies! It was wonderful! To be part of that healing ministry and to see people healed. You just can't put words on how wonderful that was. Look over there on the bookshelf, I still have the notes I took on a small pad of paper. There is the notebook, right next to the *Hunters'* book."

I get up and go to the bookshelf. Returning with the notepad, I open up to this paragraph:

> "Do all the things you've learned," Jesus tells them.
> They have to do what they've seen Jesus do.
> They go and when they come back, they are amazed at what happened!
> They come back and say to Jesus, "Wow! We were able to do this and that."
> They were very excited.

"Yeah, they really had to trust that Jesus had given them his authority," I say, after reading the notes.

"Ah, it was amazing. Some people, some very intelligent people would have said: 'This is *not* a smart move: sending us out without a cent, not a dime.' You know? 'Sending us out without an extra tunic? What if we get wet or something like that?'"

"'Aren't we supposed to be able to give some money to the poor that we meet?'"

"'Don't we have to buy bread?' But they didn't argue. It was quite amazing."

"They just did it."

"And after that, Jesus says, 'Come to the side, and come and rest with me.' And then he looks out, and there is this huge crowd, a huge crowd, and Scripture says: 'He had compassion on them.' So that's when they thought they were going to rest after all their work and effort, and they're talking to Jesus about all that had happened, and he says, now you have to feed these people. And they are thinking, hey wait a minute, we already did everything you said and now you're telling us to feed this huge crowd?"

"Right!"

"They were so obedient when he sees them out on the lake. They are fishing, they have been fishing all night and they caught nothing. And then he tells them, 'drop your nets on this other side.' They could've said: 'what do you know about fishing? Fishing's our profession and we've been here all night. Now you're asking us to drop our nets to the side? We know where the fish are usually and they're not there.' But they do it! And they had toiled all night, but then they came back with a huge catch of fish, and they are thinking, Wow!"

"It seems that when Jesus steps in, it's abundance! A huge amount."

"Yes! It doesn't just say they caught a bunch of fish."

"A huge amount. Two boats full of fish. It says the boats were almost sinking."

"And then feeding the multitudes. And there was so much of the bread and fish left over. They filled 12 baskets."

"Yeah, they probably had big baskets back then too. And then at Cana, He changes jars filled with water into the equivalent of *six hundred* one liter bottles of wine."

"Yes, like you say, it's not just enough. It's abundance!"

"So just because we can't access Dad's mind, doesn't mean that Jesus doesn't have an abundance to give him in another way!"

"That's true! He knew so many scriptures. He had sheets typed out with the Word of God that he knew by heart."

"Yeah, they are in this box where he keeps his Bible. Look at this fine print. Six cards with scriptures on both sides."

"Now, the way things are, I am not sure *what* he knows," my mother says with concern.

"Let's pray," I answer, asking the Lord for help with my dad. Then I pray for my mom's colon to keep healing.

"You know, Marc, I am feeling stronger, and not as tired. Thank you for your prayers and for all you are doing with Dad."

"I am glad you feel better, Mom. One thing is for sure about Dad. Jesus can heal him, Jesus wants to heal him, and Jesus will heal him. We'll find a way to reach his heart," I say.

"Hope so, for Dad's sake. Well, thank you Marc, for doing laundry. Dad is sleeping in clean pajamas tonight."

FREEDOM FROM THE VORTEX

E ven with the progress I have made, things now start to get worse. My Dad becomes more and more aggressive. When it comes time to go to the bathroom, he grips his belt with his hands and will not let me take his pants down. I'm sorry to put it this way, but he holds on to his pants with as much vehemence and determination as if he is afraid that he will be violated.

Every single time is the same. I ask myself over and over: *What happened when he spent that year in an all-boys school in England?* Is this touching on a nerve that requires healing?

When my Mom tries taking his pants down, he grabs both her wrists, squeezing them hurtfully and not letting them go despite her pleas. He refuses to take down his pants himself.

When I am with him and my father grips his pants, his muscular strength becomes superhuman. Stronger than me. I cannot physically override my Dad by forcing him to take down his pants. I know that to try would be a BIG MISTAKE.

The frustration is intense for me when he starts holding on and won't let go. I feel almost compelled to use force. I have scenes in my mind from movies where at the sound of a buzzer, two tough, burly big wardens come in and manhandle the man who is resisting them, forcing him to submit to the very thing he fears — being undressed against his will.

I always hate when this happens. Choosing to dominate by force is a misuse of authority when it concerns a basically helpless person. This kind of behavior is not normal. Our medical world tries to control it with meds, solitary confinement, etc. From His perspective, Jesus sees a man possessed by or acting under the power of an evil spirit. To use human force in this kind of struggle only ends up being harmful, and creates accompanying feelings of isolation, powerlessness, and resentment. Worst of all, it helps the devil-disease-dictatorship accomplish its goal of separation, alienation, and estrangement.

My Dad needs to be valued. He needs to be treated with respect and validated, and yet this struggle is pushing me to use force against him.

The frustration keeps mounting. I am scrambling for some kind of control in the midst of feeling overcome by his superhuman strength.

At the point of near violence, I hear a firm voice:

"Back OFF. Just back off!"

This isn't my voice. Or my dad's voice! Or my mom's voice.

I hear these words as a clear command from the Lord. This is an order given to me, as firm and as strong as I have ever heard the Lord Jesus speak to me.

"OK, I'll stand in the doorway," I say.

What a relief to feel that I have the power to let go and back up to the doorway of the bathroom.

This is the voice of prudence and I hear it loud and clear. How much the Alzheimer's devil-dictator-disease wants to sabotage all our progress! I will not let that happen and am very grateful and relieved to receive such a command, straight from the Commander-in-Chief of the Heavenly Armies.

"Step back!" He says.

"Yes, Lord."

Only as I step back, do I break clean from being sucked into the infernal vortex of the deadly tornado, bidding me to tangle and twist and wrestle and curse and cry out: "What is wrong with you?"

and raise my voice in frustration at a poor human being who is now under the influence of an evil spirit.

I back off each and every time Jesus tells me to. It is clear that I am not fighting my father's own weak flesh and muscle strength, but rather the power of evil spirits trying to take over his flesh and muscle strength. The evil spirits' demonic influence over him manifests in my father having either a mocking or a defiant spirit toward me, all the while holding out against me with super-human strength.

From my new vantage point in the doorway of the bathroom, it is clear that I need to command the evil spirits to depart. I don't need the Lord to speak to me again about this next move. I am well aware of the Holy Spirit's presence here and of the new authority I have from this position. "For though we walk in the flesh, we do not war after the flesh." (2 Corinthians 10:3 NKJ).

I must add a side note to these events. Some people believe that we are to *ask* the Lord to get rid of the devil, or that only a priest or a minister can do this. Actually, Jesus gave his disciples and He has given all believers the authority to get rid of the devil. It is up to us.

"And He said to them, 'I saw Satan fall like lightning from heaven. I have given you the authority to trample on serpents and scorpions, and over all the power of the enemy, and nothing shall by any means hurt you. Nevertheless, do not rejoice in this, that the spirits are subject to you, but rather rejoice because your names are written in heaven.'" (Luke 10:18-20 NKJ).

My commands are tentative at first, but they still work, and I become more confident. I say:

"Depart right now you evil spirit of mockery. Depart right now you evil spirit of defiance. Get out of here in the name of Jesus, by the blood of Jesus and by the cross of Jesus." I stand up to the evil spirit using "the weapons of our warfare which are not carnal, but mighty through God to the pulling down of strong holds." (2 Corinthians. 10:4 NKJ)

I do not need to shout. My father doesn't need to hear me speak in a way that scares him. I speak the command quietly, but with authority, knowing that it is the authority that counts. Any loud volume would confuse my father.

However, the evil spirits are extremely persistent, which pushes me to my limits it seems — but God's grace is always there, seeing me through. As far as my dream of reaching his heart, where did that go?

I do feel like I am on the right track all the same, because I am definitely acting in non-violent defiance of the dictatorship's regime. To confront true evil at first is exhausting though, and, to give you an idea, after 90 minutes of standing up to it, I feel like I have worked a full day of washing and detailing cars.

These assaults become less exhausting to confront as I learn to back off physically and emotionally; having done so, I immediately find rest.

The test, I know, to determine the reality of the situation, is simply to command the evil spirit to depart and — if it is an evil spirit — it will be gone, and I will instantly see a change in my father. I can casually re-enter the bathroom, after casting out the evil spirit, and start over.

"Hey, Dad! Good to see you!" I say slowly as if I am talking to a child. "Okay, it's time to go to the bathroom. So, I am going to loosen your belt and lower your pants. OK, go ahead; you can sit down on the toilet."

These words meet with...no resistance! My touching his belt provokes no reaction *at all* on his part. The change is like flicking a switch. On/Off. Night and Day.

In the time it takes to speak a simple command, we go from contentious torment to restful grace. Amazing difference.

Amazing Grace.

My father is docile as a lamb and yields to grace like a little lamb in my hands. 'The Lord's sheep,' my mother calls him.

So now in this bathroom with the pretty porcelain sink painted with flowers and the big mirror behind it, there's a very friendly and welcoming space. The Lord is here.

In no time my father's pants are dropped and my father is sitting on the toilet seat, taking care of business with an air of contentment. Then when he is done, yes, there is still the clean-up, but it is accomplished with ease.

"My yoke is easy," is the phrase our Lord Jesus uses to describe the amazing benefits we reap when we live our lives in Him and He lives His life in us.

"Come to Me all you who labor and are heavy laden, and I will give you rest," Jesus says. "Take my yoke upon you, and learn from Me, for I am gentle and lowly in heart, and you will find rest for your souls. For My yoke is easy and my burden is light." (Matthew 11:30 NKJ).

Is this not the same picture of Jesus that we see in the Gospels? When Jesus speaks "Peace" to the stormy seas of Lake Galilee? When he casts out a 'Legion' of evil spirits from the 'demoniac of Gerasenes,' so that the man can be healed who is living homeless and naked, completely isolated in a cemetery, and become "the man from whom the demons had departed, sitting at the feet of Jesus, clothed and in his right mind." So that afterward, Jesus can say, "Return to your own house, and tell what great things God has done for you." He can go back to his family, and tell them everything God has done for him. (Luke 8:22-39 NKJ).

This is the miracle that Jesus is doing for my father. This is the miracle that needs to happen in face of this vortex of hell, commonly called, "the anger period."

There is a 'Do Not Enter' sign on this door and it says: "Do Not Enter Without Jesus." The dictatorship of Alzheimer's is ruthless and cunning, and will chew me up and hurt my Dad and spit us out, as well as all who love him, if we try to enter the vortex of hell in our own strength.

However, I'm happy to say that we can successfully enter with Jesus. Jesus has authority over all evil spirits and Alzheimer's is no exception. Jesus is alive today and he is wonderful. "Jesus Christ is the same yesterday, today and forever." (Hebrews. 13: 8 NKJ). "For the scriptures tell us that no one who believes in Christ will ever be disappointed." (Romans. 10: 11 TLB).

The confusing part is that this is the same Dad who is still acting nice in the hallway, the bedroom, the kitchen and the living room.

How am I to feel about my father's current behavior? How am I to proceed?

This is where the training is important and also the resolve. The Lord is with me. I know He is for sure. At this point on our journey, I am all the more determined to only say positive things to my Dad.

My words are identity tags that will mark him and his future and which he has little ability to dispute, for good or for bad. Yes, I have the power of choice for him, and as it says in Proverbs 18:21: "Death and life are in the power of the tongue, and those who love it will eat its fruit." (NKJ).

I know that with Jesus's help, I don't have to give in to the negativity of the sickness. And I know that on the level of my father still hearing words of life, he doesn't have to give into it either. Just because he cannot respond to me very much, does not mean he can't hear me.

I believe he can hear me and that my words have the power to give him life, to build him up, to set him free. I want to speak positive words of life to him in the faith that he will receive them.

"Dad, you don't have to do what the sickness is telling you to do," I say. "Is this what you would normally do? OK, I am changing you. Is stepping into the bathtub what you would normally do? No way!"

Then I say: "You have to do what you would do normally. You are a child of God. Don't get distracted by all this stuff. Say: 'You evil spirit of defiance and mockery, get out of here in the name of Jesus, by the cross of Jesus and by the blood of Jesus.'"

It is both a positive statement to him and a firm command which the evil spirit will have to obey.

With my words, I can build an independent state, free from the devil-disease-dictatorship's control by leading my father to choose life and to receive God's blessing with my words. For a positive change, I need positive words.

I cannot say things like: "You are so difficult!" or "You're such a pain," or "What the?"

I try to be on the same page as my mom on this, but one day she bursts out and says: "What is wrong with you?" in frustration, after my father's latest refusal to budge.

"Well, he's got Alzheimer's. How's that for starters?" I answer in return, with my own frustrated feelings. "We have to build him up with positive words, even when he is being difficult! No matter how crazy Dad acts, he can still hear us. That is why we always have to talk positively to him. If we talk to him lovingly, maybe he will talk back to us lovingly one day."

"But Marc, Dad is not out of it!"

"This isn't exactly his normal behavior, either!"

"The Lord is a very present help in the time of trouble," says my mom after some thought. "Thank God he is not incapacitated right now. Bobby, my bear," my mom says, trailing off.

My mother worked at Hospice for years and I remind her of what she's told me several times. "Mom, you always say that people who act unresponsive can still hear, and to be careful what you say in their presence."

"That's right! It is a documented fact that hearing is the last sense to go," my mom answers emphatically. "That is why it is so important to say loving words around people who don't seem able to respond, like unconscious people on their death bed or people who are in a coma or incapacitated."

Mom is preaching to the choir.

"Amen," I say.

THE WEAPONS OF OUR WARFARE ARE MIGHTY

Twice, the authority that Jesus has given me is supremely challenged. Who am I to mess with a perfectly wrapped up deal from the devil? What authority do I really have?

"I am going to kill you," my own father says to me in the hallway outside of the bathroom.

Five words said with force, requiring me to choose: do I stand down before him or do I stand up to him? Do I say: "That hurts!" or do I say: "No, you can't. You don't have that kind of power over me."

This sudden hit on my well-being happens without warning and without regard for the hundreds of hours I have spent helping him build a sense of honor and connection.

The words are spoken with my father's crime boss gritty tone of finality. But it must be said that I am protected.

His words have all the force of a close-range bullet, but I am not blown away. I feel hit fairly hard, but God's angels are close to me, to protect me and limit the hit.

Now it is time for me to use my authority and deflect the hit and take out the enemy:

"No, you are not going to kill me! I am a child of God! I am protected by the name of Jesus Christ."

I answer fast and put up a shield to bounce that bullet right back: "I am protected by the name of Jesus Christ and He gives me power to tread upon all the power of the enemy, so you have no power over me by the blood of Jesus. Furthermore, God promises me long life for honoring my parents, which is what I am doing with you and Mom. I am here, taking care of you and honoring you, so I declare your words to be null and void by the cross of Christ!" (Ephesians. 3:2 NKJ)

That is all the firepower that I can muster, but it is enough to repel the deadly assault.

I feel back in my place, and my father stands back in turn. He goes back to being harmless, says nothing, looks sober and like he has just checked into a new place, and he is surprised to see me here. I am almost expecting him to say: "When did you get here?"

Though he seems sober in this moment of awareness, I don't feel cozy with him or that it is time to celebrate. I am still getting over the trauma of the impact. Yes, I countered his words with the Word of God, so I feel victorious, but exhausted, nonetheless.

The second direct confrontation takes place that same week, in exactly the same location in the hallway by the bathroom.

He nonchalantly approaches me and says this fragment of a sentence, with the same crime boss tone: "What you will be able to do in your short life," with a bitter, disdaining tone on *short life*.

Now that makes me mad.

Short life! I think. *That is not going to happen!*

"Short life!" I say. "That is not going to happen! I will live and not die. Furthermore, I refuse those words of intimidation, in the name of Jesus Christ. I will have a long life. God has promised me a long life for honoring my parents, which is what I am doing with you and Mom. By the cross of Jesus, be gone Satan, depart right now and take all your buddy evil spirits with you to the pits of hell. I am going to be with Jesus forever, sitting with him at his banquet table. Satan, you are going to be in the lake of fire for all eternity, so why don't you just go there right now, by the blood of Jesus, the name of Jesus and the cross of Jesus." (Revelation 20:10 NKJ).

My rebuke works and whatever evil is motivating my father instantly drops, and disappears. He seems 'normal' again.

When I see him, it is still hard to distinguish whether my dad's words are spoken by either an evil spirit or by Satan, since here is Bob, my father, in the hallway, looking pretty much the same as usual. He looks harmless, yet wasn't he aiming to take me down two minutes ago? Wasn't that him, pronouncing his pointed verdict over my life, as a gritty, tough guy with a contract out to get me?

These two events shake me up, but they do signal a final end to this period of demonic warfare, as the obstinate evil spirits lose their hold more and more on my father — and on me! My father becomes more responsive and more alive; I can talk to him and he responds.

What I have come to realize is that the evil spirits have been the fierce guardians of the Alzheimer's-dictatorship-disease. They stand at the gates, armed and ready to fight all travelers who show up with a visa to the heart. They represent the military power of the dictatorship and believe their use of force will guarantee the on-going rule of the disease-dictatorship.

The violence the evil spirits try to provoke in my mother and I during this "Anger Period" has the same evil goal of the dictatorship — to annihilate, destroy, isolate, humiliate and discourage all persons trying to rescue my father.

All my well-meaning efforts do nothing in the face of this military might. Humanly speaking and in my own strength, I am facing a power much stronger than myself. To try to defeat this evil in my own strength, without the authority given to me by Jesus to make the evil spirits depart, will result in more harm and failure.

"Unless the Lord builds the house, they labor in vain who build it." (Psalm 127:1 NKJ).

The Good News is that I am *not* on my own. I have a Savior who is stronger than every evil spirit and can make them leave, and restore every tormented soul to be: "sitting at the feet of Jesus, clothed and in their right mind." (Luke 8:35 NKJ).

The Good News is this: "For though we walk in the flesh, we do not war according to the flesh. For the weapons of our warfare are not carnal (flesh and blood, our own human strength) but mighty in God for pulling down strongholds, casting down arguments and every high thing that exalts itself against the knowledge of God, bringing every thought into captivity to the obedience of Christ." (2 Corinthians 10:3-5 NKJ). "Our fight is not against flesh and blood — but against principalities and powers of darkness in high places." (2 Corinthians 10:4 TLB).

This is why we use God's weapons of warfare, starting with the cross.

Through the ages of church history, the cross was, is, and always will be the most effective of God's weapons to make the enemy take flight.

Joan of Arc, the heroine and saint of France, upon approaching the English before her first battle had a vision of the cross upon which Christ was crucified. The voice which spoke to her said: *By this sign, you shall succeed.* Subsequently, she led the tattered and tired army of France to victory, after they had been losing ground to the British for almost one hundred years.

The power of the cross is reiterated in Colossians 2:15, where it says that Jesus disarmed the principalities and powers of darkness through his cross. "And you being dead in your trespasses...He has made alive together with Him, having forgiven you all trespasses, having wiped out the handwriting of requirements that was against us, which was contrary to us. And he has taken it out of the way, having nailed it to the cross. Having disarmed principalities and powers, He made a public spectacle of them, triumphing over them in it." (Colossians 2:15 NKJ).

"Making a public spectacle of them" is what a Roman conqueror did. The Lord Jesus is that conqueror, leading his victory procession, with the enemy in tow behind him. The enemy is Satan, now stripped of his power — the power of death and hell — naked and in chains, defeated, without weapons, and plainly shown openly to the whole world to be the coward and criminal atrocity that he is.

Jesus conquered the devil and his works through his cross. Jesus came to heal and deliver all who are under the power of the devil. Acts 10: 38 says, "God anointed Jesus of Nazareth with the Holy Spirit and with power, who went about doing good and healing all who were oppressed by the devil, for God was with Him." (NKJ)

So when we are dealing with warfare and we have mighty weapons through God, we must use them.

"By the sign of the cross, you shall succeed," was the promise made to Joan of Arc. The promise is true for all of us.

On the cross, Jesus died in our place for the remission of our sins and took the punishment we deserve so that we can be declared righteous, and be restored to the love of the Father and have eternal life.

The cross embodies the Name of Jesus and the Blood of Jesus. The name of Jesus is used repeatedly in the Acts of the Apostles as the power to bring about healing. The blood of Jesus redeems us from sin, Satan, and death.

Derek Prince, famous for his Ministry of Deliverance from evil spirits, calls the blood of Jesus "God's atomic weapon." On his Ministry prayer card entitled "God's atomic weapon," Derek Prince writes about what the blood of Jesus does for us:

> *"Through the blood of Jesus, we are redeemed out of the hand of the devil and all our sins are forgiven. Satan has no place in us, no power over us, through the blood of Jesus."*

THE HEALING MINISTRY

O n Sundays, I start going to All Saints Episcopal Church, which is three blocks walk from my mom and dad's apartment.

I begin going there after being invited by a lady named Barbara Ball whom I meet in Stein Mart during one of my rare outings. I mention to her that she is wearing a beautiful cross and after exchanging a few stories, we soon become fast friends.

She is in her 80's but has a youthful quality and a spunkiness that I find refreshing. Her husband, Howard, is strong and healthy in contrast to my Dad. I love her sense of humor; she tells people that I "picked her up at Stein Mart."

Associated with All Saints, I come to find out, is the Healing Ministry of All Saints, located in a big old house on the church grounds, called the Glennon House. The house has been restored to good condition and converted to a house of prayer and healing.

Naturally, I begin going there whenever I am able, and as God would have it, I talk with a pastor named Steve for an hour. During our relaxing time together, which comes about because of a canceled appointment, I share about casting out the evil spirits that have taken hold of my dad.

"Where did you learn about that stuff?" he asks me. "Very few people want to mess with casting out evil spirits. The pastors here at the church stay away from it."

I tell him about the man who made the most impact on my life, my spiritual father, Dr. T.L. Osborn. I tell him about Dr. T.L.

Osborn's healing ministry, which reached hundreds of thousands of people, during his overseas crusades. These Crusades have been in action for 50 years, in 100 countries. Steve talks with me about his mentor and friend, Fr. Al Durrance, who is very comfortable rebuking evil spirits. We also talk about the healing ministry of Dr. Francis McNutt and the significance of his book "Deliverance from Evil Spirits." At one point, Pastor Steve jumps up, goes into the office, and returns with two small square sheets of paper which he hands to me.

"Here, Marc," he says. "Say these prayers as often as you need. They will help you. I have found them to be extremely helpful in the healing and deliverance ministry."

"Thank you, Pastor Steve. God bless you!"

What a great visit. Now I am equipped with the two small sheets of paper that I guard carefully and read often.

The prayers talk about breaking the power of hexes, spells, and curses and rendering them null and void. This is when I start to realize that my father, and consequently my mother, have undoubtedly been under a curse my whole life.

This curse put my Dad in bondage.

My Dad became subject to the workings of evil spirits when his own mother subjected him to her evil affair with another man, while his own father was still alive. And it is no coincidence that she lived in Connecticut, near Hartford, a historical place where where actual witches practiced their abominable behavior, and the location of the first American witch hunt. As a child, I felt repelled by the very spirit of her lust.

So, I start breaking the power of all the hexes, curses and spells that could have ever been spoken over me, and over my father and mother. I go to the Healing Service for breaking Generational curses, which Pastor Steve leads in the church.

The curse ultimately does breaks off of my father, thank God, as we shall see.

Here are the prayers, unabridged, for your benefit. I highly recommend them to you.

A Prayer for Protection by Dr. Francis MacNutt
(To be prayed before ministry)

In the Name of Jesus Christ and by the power of his Cross and his Blood, we bind up the power of all evil spirits and command them not to block our prayers. We bind up the powers of earth, air, water, fire, the netherworld and the satanic forces of nature.

We break all curses, hexes and spells spoken against us and declare them null and void. We break the assignments of all evil spirits sent against us and send them to Jesus to deal with them as he will. Lord, we ask you to bless our enemies by sending your Holy Spirit to lead them to repentance and conversion.

Furthermore, we bind all interaction and communication in the world of evil spirits as it affects us and our ministry.

We ask for the protection of the shed blood of Jesus Christ over_____. Thank you, Lord, for your protection and send your Angels, especially Saint Michael, the Archangel, to help us in the battle. We ask you to guide us in our prayers: share with us your Holy Spirit's power and compassion. Amen.

Prayer to Be Set Free by Dr. Francis McNutt
(To be prayed following ministry)

Lord Jesus, thank you for sharing with us your wonderful ministry of healing and deliverance. Thank you for the healings we have seen and experienced today.

We realize that the sickness and evil we encounter is more than our humanity can bear, so cleanse us of all sadness, negativity or despair that we may have picked up. If our ministry has tempted us to anger, impatience or lust, cleanse us of those temptations and replace them with love, joy and peace.

All evil spirits that have attached themselves to us or oppressed us in any way we command you to depart — now — and go straight to Jesus Christ for him to deal with you as he will.

Come Holy Spirit: renew us, fill us anew with your power, your life, and your joy. Strengthen us where we have felt weak and clothe us with your strength. Fill us with life. Lord Jesus, please send your holy angels to minister to us and our families — guard us and protect us from all sickness, harm, and accidents.

We praise you now and forever, Father, Son, and Holy Spirit, and we ask these things in Jesus' holy Name that he may be glorified. Amen.

MOUNTAIN CLIMBING

Even as the evil spirits are trying to hold on to my dad, I start planning to change gears and add a new element.

In order to establish an independent state in him, it is time to find a positive, life-giving activity that I can do with my father, to focus my father on the positive part of his life. It's time to get my father in touch with what gives him meaning and purpose.

It's time to reach his heart.

During the evenings after Dad is in bed, I sit with my mom on the white couch in the back of the living room. Behind the couch is a row of large windows facing north. The view reveals mostly a night sky which can only be perceived with the lights off in the room. Various lamps in the apartment are turned on before dinner time and the result creates a quaint feeling.

My Mom profits from this time by reading one of her favorite books. She loves *Into Thin Air* by Jon Krakauer; the book involves a climb that goes terribly wrong on Mount Everest, a mountain climbed by friends of hers, not involved in that tragedy.

I sit to her left, next to her for a while, mainly as a gesture of solidarity since we both have our challenges with Bob and this is a time of rest.

On the wall to the right of the couch is a huge bookshelf full of the same books that I grew up with in Paris. When my father returned to the States after being in France for 12 years, the management consulting company he worked for had paid for the move.

This always seemed to me like an enormous amount of weight for them to be taking across the Atlantic, and I always figured the move must have cost them a fortune.

Whenever I ask my mom about the weight, she casually says,

"No, they were very gracious about it. The only comment I heard was, 'That was quite a heavy load you brought back.'"

Some nights I invariably rummage through the shelves in search of an appealing book to read. One evening, while my mother is reading *Into Thin Air,* I find another book about climbing mountains. It is written by Lionel Terray, a famous French guide, who made a lifetime out of climbing mountains all over the world.

To my delight it is in French; French is still my native heart language. The 5" x 8" hardcover book on the subject of mountain climbing is documented with black and white photographs.

From the moment I start reading, I really enjoy the writing. Lionel Terray is extremely articulate; he is almost a poet, which creates a sense of wonder in me, all the more since mountain climbing isn't exactly one of the literary arts.

What strikes me is that being a guide is a real passion for him — as is writing, which I can relate to. Certainly, he is writing as a means of self-expression, and also in the end, as a means of letting the world know the profound meaning of his experience.

From the outset, his title captivates me: *LES CONQUERANTS DE L'INUTILE/2,* which translates as *The Conquerors of the Useless/2.*

I come across several passages which interest me and inspire me, especially since I have been exposed to mountain climbing for years.

From a young age, my parents had taken me and my younger brother up the hiking trails of many mountains, in the Swiss Alps and in the French Pyrenees. They loved hiking those trails. My mother had climbed with her beloved father on mountains since she was a young girl.

Climbing the Matterhorn was one of my parents' most fulfilling achievements. A now-yellowed montage of photos from the climb faces my bed; in the pictures, taken by their guide, my parents are smiling triumphantly at the summit of the formidable mountain.

My father passionately wanted to teach us rock climbing when we were growing up, and coincidentally one hour from where we lived in Paris, laid the grand estate of Fontainebleau.

After a preliminary walk we came upon a huge forest — not made of trees — but of adjoining boulders and rocks, stretched out as far as the eye could see.

They were perfect climbing rocks, and I loved the challenge of scaling up the rock face, finding even the smallest foot holds and hand holds; I remember the daring challenge it posed to jump from one big, high rock to the other, and the thrill I experienced upon landing.

Keeping in mind my humble yet rewarding adventures in rock climbing, I am inspired by Lionel Terray's insights into his work as a mountain guide. Here is my favorite passage, translated by yours truly from French to English:

My Work as a Guide
by Lionel Terray

"I will say again that, without exception, the work of a guide does not consist of pulling off exploits, but in taking the classic climbs and the easy trails — and I would be at fault to complain about this fact.

For that matter, even in the most modest realizations, this work has never ceased to evoke a passion in me.

Almost always, between the guide and his client, a symbiotic state is created which, in this profession, gives to all human relations an atmosphere which is more agreeable than all others.

Giving to a client the joy of climbing a peak, a peak that without you he would have never been able to attain, has always seemed to me like a work of creation. Such a hands-on achievement makes me feel the same pleasure that a craftsman has in fashioning a work of art he loves, or that an artist has in producing a masterpiece."
(*The Conquerors of the Useless/2*, p. 37)

Lionel's commentary sparks some inspiring ideas in me. After saying good night to my mother, I head straight for my journal and write the following reflection on the role of a guide:

My Journal Entry:

Reflections on the role of the Guide after reading *The Conquerors of the Useless/2*.

Climbing is exhilarating. It is good exercise, physically and mentally challenging, requiring both nerve and agility. On the mountain climbs, you go from the base camp up a trail to the foot of the mountain. The air is invigorating and there is a great sense of achievement, of freedom and of conquering the little fears that stop you from doing something big.

For this journey has a goal: to go beyond what you consider to be impossible to accomplish to a place you never dreamed possible. Hurts from being abused, the immobility of depression are parts of your past you will look down on in the same way as you will gaze upon the clouds from the mountain peak.

But who will lead the way up the trail? Where is the trail? Is it up to us to find it? Do we have the ability to make it on our own?

Many have gone before us. Take comfort in this thought: with each challenge the world has faced, there has been a record breaker. The four-minute mile. The Everest. The truth is that to go beyond ourselves, we need someone to guide us. Someone who has gone before us, who has been there. We need a guide. Having a guide means we are no longer alone. There is someone who will accompany us and be at our side.

The gift of the guide is that he will enable us to do what we could never do for ourselves in a million years. Because we are all handicapped in some way, we are prevented from going the distance without a helping hand when we arrive at that crucial junction. There will be that one part of the climb too hard to do on our own without help from the guide. Without completing that crossing, we will never know the joy of making it to the top.

For several dinners to come, I ask my mom to tell me more about her beloved father.

My mom has the highest admiration for her father. Besides talking about Cillery, my mom shares inspiring stories about what it was like to live with her father in a third-floor apartment in Lyon, two floors below an apartment the Gestapo had taken by force, evicting and arresting the Jewish family that lived there during WWII.

My French grandfather was a war hero. He could not give in to a foreign invader taking away the liberty and lifestyle his countrymen had worked so hard to accomplish for France, the country they all loved. He fought in two world wars, making three daring escapes from the German army. He would not give up the fight.

He formed an underground network for young men to escape the grasp of the Nazis as they went through occupied France, seizing every able bodied man to send to their Nazi factories in Germany.

Through his connections and friends over the years, he found guides to lead the men out of France, through the mountains of the Pyrenees and into Spain. From there, they made for the nearest port and boarded vessels bound for North Africa, for Morocco, where they would rejoin La France Libre, the Free French forces.

My grandfather knew the value of a guide to protect his young men and lead them to safety. The guides helped the young men do what do what they wanted to do — escape certain death — yet could not do on their own. With a guide, they had all the strength and resolve to make the journey to freedom, and the heart to make it happen.

Thus the idea is born for a guided flight to the Matterhorn with my dad.

GUIDED INTERACTIVE VISUALIZATION EXERCISE

Up until now, nothing close to an active narrative guided approach had crossed my mind.

Yet the power of storytelling is so real and so fantastic that it changed my life. I was able to stay alive after my son Josh's death, and keep him alive inside of me, by telling our story and celebrating his life.

Storytelling reaches our hearts and gives us wings to fly. Kerry, my mentor in Toastmasters, would always say: "Information tells. Stories sell." Jimmy, another mentor in Toastmasters, would stand up as a speech evaluator and often say: "I am just going to tell you one word. Story. You need to tell a story for that speech to work." The lawyer that Anthony Hopkins plays in "Amistad" says: "I find that the man with the best story wins."

So I'm adding this up in my mind. One of my father's big lines in management consulting was: "You have to get the client to 'own it.' The client has to take responsibility for being a part of the solution."

My dad needs his own wings to fly, I am thinking. *What will inspire him the most? Something he has done that he considers a great achievement. How do I bring him into his own story?*

So far I have been the one taking the initiative. My greatest success has been in my headquarters in the bathroom where I have been able to take the lead in shaving him and use that personal space to reaffirm him and to continue trying to reach his heart.

In my efforts to do more, I try 'music therapy,' which many praise as an effective therapy, but in my case, it produces not the least noticeable effect. For my Dad at this point, it is probably one of those 'I'm left to myself again' activities. This doesn't even register on the personal presence scale or on the personal Jesus scale for him.

I need to be involved even more than I am with the shaving. And I need to bring along the best of what I've learned in order to get him more involved. I have created a personal space that has helped me become his friend by talking and reaching his heart. Now I wonder if I can build on that activity and do more to involve him, both physically and in a way that reaches him more deeply.

What if he can get back in touch with part of himself? What if he can get back in touch with his own story? Will that reach his heart?

I seriously owe my desire to attempt to unleash the power of guided visual imaging to one movie which I rented many years ago, back in 1998, and which is now hard to find, and currently available only on VHS. It is called, "Question of Faith."

This movie made a very strong impression on me. In the movie, the heroine gets set free from a place of guilt and condemnation as an old memory — in black and white — comes to light through visual imaging. Her imagination is able to bring her to a new place of freedom and healing — in color.

Most noteworthy is the unforgettable combined succession of photographic scenes, created in the interior of her imagination as she follows and is empowered by the leading of the Guide-narrator's voice. This is called Visual Guided Imagery. Most accurately, I will choose to call my experience Guided Interactive Visualization Exercise. G.I.V.E.

The difference is that the Guide in the film, "Question of Faith" is saying, "Imagine you are in a safe place."

It was up to the heroine to choose and imagine her safe place. The Guide is giving her an exercise she can do on her own, when and where she wants to, without her guide needing to be there in person.

My role as Guide with my father is to interact in an exercise together with him; all the while leading his imagination every step of the way on a journey which follows a storyline of which I am the narrator. The key is that I am physically involved with him all through the storyline.

This Guided Interactive Visualization Exercising is a narrative adventure — beginning in reality and moving into an imagined visual achievement — which is based on his greatest physical accomplishment in reality: reaching the summit of the Matterhorn.

I did not go on that climb. My father, Bob Swift successfully accomplished that arduous climb with his beloved wife, Monique.

When it came to my dad and me, we had both shared another climb — on a mountain in the Pyrenees, in a test of our determination, which proved to be the greatest physical experience of bonding between us.

My mother and brother Greg were drained and decided to hang out on a rock slab while my dad and I finished the climb to the summit.

To do this, we had to climb up and cross over a ridge and slowly trudge up a very steep snow slope. We made it to the summit and felt exhilarated.

Coming back down, we missed the ridge and found ourselves way downhill. When we looked up behind us and realized that we had missed our pass, I remember feeling very deflated and frustrated. We were already exhausted. Now we had a long way to climb back up.

I didn't get angry with my dad.

Although he was the guide and was responsible for leading the climb, I somehow felt that I shared in the responsibility of not seeing the ridge.

We slowly made the climb back up the trail, kicking our boots into the snow one footstep at a time, for what seemed like an hour for each minute. Nothing compared to the victory of reaching the ridge, crossing over and being able to go back down the right trail and back home. I don't even remember the summit, but to this day I remember each of the steps we made on that steep slope, as our hiking boots dug into the snow in an effort to get a good grip in the slippery wall towering above us and not slip back down. It took an impossibly long time for us to make it back up to the pass.

I felt I had accomplished a very great thing that day, because I did it shoulder-to-shoulder, and man-to-man with my dad.

My mom and Greg missed out on this bonding experience, and I think, wrote it off as more of an embarrassment for my father than the triumph it represented for me. To me, it was about overcoming something against all odds. Thus far, the event has not taken its place among the annals of the Swift family achievements; I am the only one who values its significance.

Now, many years later, I find myself rejoined with my father in the honorable task of conquering against all odds — "redeeming time when men think least I will," — William Shakespeare, Henry IV Part I: Act 1, Scene 2. We are both involved physically, interacting at the same time, united to attain a common goal. Ultimately, this exercise proves to circumvent his brain and accomplish our goal of reaching his heart.

Guided Interactive Visualization Exercise

Guided: I am helping him imagine that his arms are wings. I am helping him imagine that he is flying. I am leading his flight by telling a story in which we take a flight over a lake, over a forest and to the summit of the Matterhorn. The narrative awakens his senses of touch, hearing, smell, taste, and sight so that all five of his senses and his imagination are experiencing the events as he yields to and participates in my narration of the story.

Interactive: I am holding his arms, flapping them up and down, and going with him. We are involved with both of our bodies and senses. I give him the joy of the experience, pacing the movement of his wings, ending by moving his arms harder and faster and saying: "We are almost there, keep it up!"

Visualization: I am helping him to visualize an experience to which hopefully he will respond to, by tapping into the memories of the event he lived. By doing so I am putting him in touch with his feelings of success, his positive feelings of well-being and his sense of achievement.

Exercise: This is physical exercise; for him, it is gymnastics, a workout with multiple benefits! For me, it is an exercise of weight lifting and endurance.

Our daily flights to the Matterhorn grow better through repetition, each time expanding a little more — not always longer — but stronger. By now, my father is willing to follow my voice and to go with me on this adventure.

FLYING TO THE SUMMIT

Thus begins a journey which humbly grows to become a turning point in our lives.

Around three or four in the afternoon, I bring my father into the living room.

"Please come to the corner of the living room with me, Dad," I say. "Good. Now stand facing the window. I am going to stand behind you. Now look out the window."

We're looking out the window and Dad is standing with his back to me, as I stand squarely behind him.

"You see that tree out there, Dad?" I start off our journey by saying. "You see that big tree with all the branches? Now I don't know if you can make it out, but behind those branches, there is a lake. You see that bluish color between the branches? It is almost a blue-gray. Well, that's the lake. So what we are going to do is fly up to the top of the Matterhorn today. You have successfully climbed the Matterhorn with Mom and we are going to go there again today. Okay, so we're going to start off by flying over the tree and over the lake. So lift up your wings and get ready to fly!"

At this point, I lift up my Dad's arms from behind, holding them so I can flap them up and down. I let my hands rest under his arms, comfortably balancing the weight between his elbows and his wrists. Once I set that steady point, I slowly begin raising his arms.

"Okay, here we go!"

I'm adjusting my knees, holding in my stomach. I let his arms drop down and lift them up again. I begin a steady motion of arm movements, which will continue until we reach the summit of the Matterhorn.

I begin our journey.

"Okay Dad, we're flying over the tree and we are swooping down over the water. The water is right beneath us and we are flying over it. You feel that mist on your face, Dad? That's spray from the lake from the wind."

Now I imitate the sound of geese:

"Wonk, wonk, wonk!"

"Wow, Dad, that's geese. They are flying right past us."

"Wonk, wonk, wonk, wonk, wonk!"

"Hi, geese!"

We fly some more then I say: "We're reaching the edge of the lake now and we're going to fly over a big forest. Okay, that's good! Just fly up higher, up over the forest. Can you smell the pine trees?"

I keep his arms (which are now his wings) slowly moving up and down. He is flying thanks to me moving his arms and telling him that he is flying.

I have an ideal story length and it gets adjusted according to the strength in my arms as they are holding my Dad's arms and moving them up and down.

I choose this visual guided imagery and this particular journey because it represents a memorable accomplishment for my dad and my mom. It was a climb that pushed my father to the limits of his endurance and I'm journeying back to his real life climb on a solidarity mission to reaffirm and draw new life from the mass of sensory memories created by his experience.

FREE THE BODY MEMORY

Triumphing over difficulty through physical strength imprints a profound memory in the body.

The muscles themselves and the skin, the very bones and the joints, the hands and feet, the face, the head, the heart, the organs, the lungs, all join together to overcome against all odds — and they remember their achievement with a great sense of awe.

In repeating this exercise every day, my father draws from the depths of his body memory a touch of those same feelings of joy and satisfaction, and a taste of confidence, accomplishment, and peace.

It's like the stories of the heightened senses of blind people: they hear and smell and feel and taste more powerfully. So to make up for my Dad's brain that is "blind," let's get in touch with and set his body memory free.

Let's revive his body language and his body power, and activate his body energy, and give it wings to fly.

That's a great connection to live in, so I am hoping he can get lost in this journey, and re-discover this place of 'Wow, I did it!' and just be there for a while. I'm hoping he can rest in this place where he can feel good vibes inside him and be, as much as possible, intoxicated in the high again.

I want my father to have a 'now' experience, as if he really is climbing today, by activating his body memory so he can be physically engaged in an experience that is liberating to him and makes him feel in touch with himself.

My dad had been a dedicated long distance runner and jogger, running 2 to 3 miles a day. Whether he was at home or abroad, he would always faithfully set out on his run in the mornings. He liked "going the distance," and he enjoyed the sense of physical achievement, and the high created in his body by the release of the endorphins.

That is why I like the idea of helping him fly to the summit of the Matterhorn. It is an epic adventure. We can 'go the distance' and we can relive the 'impossible.' We can 'go to the top.'

Here is a short synopsis I wrote of the mountain my father and mother have successfully climbed:

The Matterhorn

To give you an idea of its magnitude, this mountain was so feared by alpinists that it was not successfully climbed until 1863. The hike to the base of the mountain is daunting — hiking around the base is a ten-day adventure.

With four steep faces of rock facing the four compass points, comes a choice of four ridges to reach the summit. These ridges are narrow, and the ascent involves negotiating a series of steps upward on jagged rocks and snow-covered paths, always flanked on both sides by a towering precipice. The summit itself is narrow and the descent extremely difficult, as the fear of falling from the dizzying heights never lets up.

The first ascent was marked by the deaths of four men, including the French Guide, Michel Croz. This disastrous event happened as one of the inexperienced climbers, Hadow, fell on the guide and knocked him over. The weight of the falling men pulled the two men above them, Hudson and Douglas, in a drag down the North face. Edward Whymper and the father and son Tangwolders, still hanging above them, were left alive when the rope broke, thanks to a sharp edge of rock the rope was laying over. By a miracle they had employed it by mistake as it was the weakest of the three ropes they had brought.

It is said this disaster put an end to the Golden Age of Alpinism, and gave all future climbers of the Matterhorn the warning to approach it with the utmost respect. Climate conditions further increased the challenge of the climb. The mountain's isolated position made it subject to rapid weather changes, banner clouds around the Matterhorn's 14,692 ft. peak, along with strong winds and storms which set in motion treacherous rock falls.

For my flight with my father, I am replicating the relatively good weather conditions which Robert, Monique, and their Guide experienced as they successfully ascended to the summit.

This takes us forward to our current flight over the forest, which is getting ever closer to the foot of the Matterhorn.

"Okay Dad, we are coming up to the base of the Matterhorn. We are flying over the base camp and we are headed up. Okay Dad, we're starting up the mountain. We are going to veer to the left here. Very good."

I'm holding his wings. It's getting tiring, but I'm putting more energy into the motion for us to fly up the face of the mountain.

"Okay Dad, we're going to traverse. Back to the right now and up that slope. Good. Now we have to cross over to the left again. Okay, now back over to the right."

By now, my arms are getting tired. My arms are — burning — would be a better way to say it. I put that energy into a sort of pain-boosted charge.

"Okay Dad. Now we have to get over this overhang. Come on. You can do it. Just make a little more effort. We're almost there. Keep going. Okay, there's the summit. I can see it. You see that rock at the top? Okay, keep going. Land there. Just a little more effort," I say, giving my dad's wings their final lift before landing on the rock.

"Okay, you did it! You landed on the rock. Well done!"

Now I gently remove my hands from under his forearms and I let go of his wings.

"Look around at all the other mountains beneath us. It is so clear and beautiful up here. Breathe Dad! Take deep breaths in and out. Breathe in and out. That's it. Good, Dad!"

Our routine develops more and more over time.

The better I can make it, the sweeter it gets. Our repeated flights progress to deeper levels of well-being, even as opposition is growing toward doing the routine things. At key moments during the day when I am close to him, he either sounds upset about getting something wrong, or becomes determined to take decisive action against "those bastards" and "wipe them out."

As I sense unresolved issues in him, guilt, regrets, and anger, I take his achievement at reaching the summit of the Matterhorn and make it a time of freeing himself from the loads he has been carrying. That is Jesus's specialty.

Then it dawns on me to have Jesus there to help him. Jesus proclaimed His mission statement when he said, "The Spirit of the LORD is upon Me, because He has anointed Me to preach the gospel to the poor; He has sent Me to heal the brokenhearted, to proclaim liberty to the captives, and recovery of sight to the blind, to set at liberty those who are oppressed; to proclaim the acceptable year of the LORD." (Luke 4:18-19 NKJ). See the extended version from which Jesus spoke in Isaiah 61:1-2a, stopping halfway because He came to save and did not come for vengeance.

"Look Dad! Jesus is here, he's been waiting for you. He went ahead of you to prepare the way."

With Jesus present at his arrival, this matter (no pun intended) is facilitated greatly. The living Jesus is delighted to be a part of our assembly. Jesus loves to be invited and welcomed. Of course, in all I am doing with my dad — sitting him down, getting him to stand up, the shaving in the bathroom, building him up with positive words, reaffirming his identity as the Father's beloved son with scriptures, cleaning and dressing him, undressing him, casting out evil spirits of mockery and defiance — I ask Jesus to be with me and am counting on Jesus to help me. Now that we are here, on the Matterhorn mountaintop, the difference is that my dad's experiential belief in this reality empowers him to act for himself.

"Dad you're here at the top. You can let that stuff go. It's okay. Let it go. Just leave it all with Jesus here on the mountaintop. He's going to fix everything. Breathe it out. Breathe in and breathe it out."

My father breathes more deeply and seems to be letting things go. He is allowing this experience to transform him into a more meditative state. To be with him is wonderful, as he effectively breathes in the fresh air of his new accomplishment and breathes out the bad stuff of his past. It is the culmination of our exercise, and his letting go achieves a marvelous sense of relief on several occasions.

MISSION OF MERCY

O ne day, as we are making headway with our flights to the Matterhorn, my Dad becomes combative and challenges me to a fight right there in the bathroom.

All the stories I read came back to me, from teachers saying how important it is to set the standard on the first day of class. I am determined to show him that I am the stronger one, and settle it once and for all.

We wrestle back and forth, but he has met his match in me. I pin both his arms against the wall and lean against him with all my weight. "Don't you ever try that again," I tell him. "I'm much stronger than you, Dad. And I will always be stronger than you. You got it?"

He does get it. The incident never happens again.

But it does do one thing that is much more positive than negative. It levels the playing field and puts us on an equal footing. Having to repeatedly keep my mind in a positive mind frame leads me to this place of a one-on-one meeting with my father over a huge unresolved issue between us.

I had a brain tumor operation at the age of 19 which almost killed me. My father had never even put his arm around me and told me that he was sorry I went through that. He had not shown me any compassion or caring that I could remember. Not once did we even have a conversation about what happened. All I could remember was that he seemed very put out and upset with me that I had wrecked his sailing vacation to the British Virgin Islands — as if having all my locks shaved off and my head cut open was something I had deliberately set out to do, to inconvenience him. To have a brain tumor at age 19 was not in my playbook.

My son Josh had shown me such compassion after our relationship began healing. He felt the pain with me and his great caring sponged up my pain. I was still very grateful for Josh's compassion and healing love.

The issue with my dad began when I was twelve. He wanted me to go to Yale like him, but we were living in Paris so he asked me to trust him and go to a British boarding school so I could learn English at the level where I would be accepted at Yale. Off I went to one of the 'best' schools in England. To him, it might've been a good idea in theory, but in practice the living conditions were so deplorably different from living in Paris that I had a very hard time adjusting. 'Nice, tidy squalor' might be good words to describe the condition of Whitelaw House in 1971, where 70 boys lived in dormitories, or how about the Biblical term, 'a haunt of demons?' Pornographic magazines were passed on in place of relationships with the opposite sex causing me both confusion and hatred for the prison I had agreed to live in. It's well-known that the French and the British have been at odds and being American was the icing on the cake. I was bullied, ridiculed and called various unsavory names.

I missed out on so many things I was looking forward to. After being with the beautiful girls in Paris, I was looking forward to dating and spending my teen years in the company of both girls and boys. In England, I spent eight months a year with only boys and no parental upbringing.

I tried to get attention by breaking rules and defying boundaries, but somehow, neither my mom nor my dad, got the message that I was very unhappy there. To make matters worse, my father started calling me a "screw up" after two years in England, even though I was doing well academically. I did so well that I got an 'A' in the French A Levels at the age of fifteen, and was accepted at both Yale and Brown. Ironically, I went to Brown and I am glad I did because I could handle the course load and graduate — even though once in college in America, my health got worse and worse. I ended up undergoing a brain tumor operation the summer of my freshman year. I was given five years to live. In the face of death, I cried out to the Lord to help me.

Jesus healed my brain two years later, and I lived. I became an on-fire Christian. Still, my parents did not want to talk about what happened or help me deal with it.

Now here I am with a father who seems out of it, yet somehow I know I will be able to talk to him about all these things that have gone wrong in my life because I am sharing with him something awfully huge that has gone wrong in his life.

Part of me did everything in my life to prove to him I wasn't a "screw up". But just at the point where I can finally show him my achievements, he looks like he is no longer there to hear me, no longer there apparently to respond with any sense of accountability, or to acknowledge my achievements and be able to say: "I'm sorry that I said that about you. You really did well."

No, at this juncture my Dad is in a: 'I'm not there,' bordering on 'I'm gone' zone, where he just seems vacant a lot of the time, and here I am, needing desperately to get some kind of response from him, even though he can't write his own name, or even make the x's and the o's to play tic tac toe.

Had I trained myself for revenge, *Count of Monte Cristo* style, this would have been my hour. But I am compelled to care for him because it has become clear that he has been living under a curse, a curse that messed us all up. I take advantage of this opportunity to talk with him, to level the playing field and deal with what has happened.

Did my father end up here because that was the best that he could do? Did all of what he put aside, and not deal with, catch up with him?

There is one truth at the basis of the teachings at the School for Spiritual Directors, held at the Pecos Benedictine Abbey in Pecos, New Mexico. I completed the program after being healed from the brain tumor in 1980. This is the truth I learned:

If you don't deal with it, it will deal with you.

The battle to deal with what happened is much more complicated than it first appears. Even my mom denies that there has been any kind of curse on our family. How am I now to fight for the heart of my father?

Yes, indeed and unfortunately she still denies this, in spite of the long list which I present to her, of failed marriages and failed parenting, of the messed up lives, divorces and deadly diseases that plague our family, and my troubled life at the British boarding school, then ending up with having five epileptic seizures and a brain tumor the size of a baseball in my head.

Whatever could be interpreted as success is always accompanied by sorrow. These events played out more like curses than blessings from God.

Psalm 91 says that when we make the Lord our refuge, even the Most High our dwelling place, no evil shall befall us, for He gives His angels charge over us to keep us in all our ways:

"A thousand may fall at your side,
And ten thousand at your right hand;
But it shall not come near you.
Only with your eyes shall you look,
And see the reward of the wicked.
Because you have made the LORD who is my refuge,

Even the Most High, your dwelling place,
No evil shall befall you,
Nor shall any plague come near your dwelling;
For He shall give His angels charge over you,
To keep you in all your ways." (Psalm 91: 7-11 NKJ)

Even if my mother cannot see that evil did befall us and that a plague did come near our dwelling, I am living witness of this truth. Even if she does not want to see that we lived under a curse, I am here. By now it is humbly evident to me that God has brought me here to salvage from destruction the end of my father's life because I am specifically equipped for this battle against the tyranny of this devil-dictatorship-Alzheimer's disease.

And to find a way to gain back the heart and the soul of my Dad. Now I am ready to give healing, not require justice, to show mercy not settle a score, to lift up, build up, and set him free. I cannot leave for dead my own father, who is now in the power of my hand and I hope, in the power of the Lord.

The moments of frustration, in dealing with his resistance to me, cause trigger points of anger that in a 'comfortable,' 'civilized' and 'proper' household might only be skimmed over by dismissive apologies with no change of heart, such as: "Yes, I'm terribly sorry that happened to you. I had no idea it was so difficult for you."

But face-to-face with my father's demanding behavior I am seeking a sense of accountability, even recognition from him. Here is my journal entry of this one explosive moment of man-to-man confrontation.

> *My Journal Entry*
> This very day, during our morning time in the bathroom, I said what rose up inside of me. This expression was prompted by what I felt like was a good reason: 'If you are pushing me to the place where I have to look at your

nudity and clean you up over and over and have to be this close to you, you're also going to hear what I have to say to you.' And off I went.

"If you had not stuck me in that sick British boarding school, I would've never ended up with horrible seizures and a brain tumor and had my life almost destroyed. I thought you cared about me. How could you make Yale so important that it almost cost me my life? If Jesus hadn't saved me, I would have died!"

Naturally or miraculously, I am not sure which, I do reach my father.

When I speak to him, using the aforementioned words to express my feelings, he hears me. I can see it by the look in his eyes.

We somehow make our way out of the bathroom and go directly across the hall, into my 'room.' He is hunched over, and his eyes look as big as saucers. In them, I see all the feelings that I, for much of my life, have longed to receive.

I can see in his heartfelt gaze redness in his eyes, a swelling, a wetness on his eyelids, close to a flow of tears, telling me that he is deeply moved.

He is taking into consideration the full weight of my soul's expression, and he seems to be realizing the damage that his actions have caused me.

Clearly, my father feels, at this moment, a deep sense of sorrow resulting in a deep sense of compassion.

Then he speaks. Not his usual words which are often off target or contrary, but words which are so powerfully real that they reach me in a very personal way.

He says: "That completely changed your life. That was worse than anyone could imagine."

The words he says might not come across as life-changing at all to someone who hasn't lived with his habitual distanced posture. Let me explain more why his comment is life changing, as it might not be clear: Never in my father's life has he shown me compassion. Now, he has Alzheimer's and by all standards he should be showing mental detachment, withdrawal, lack of recognition. So how come I can feel caring and warmth from him and in his words? They are words that he deeply means from his heart. He is speaking from his heart and it completely catches me off guard. The gritty crime boss tough guy is gone a million miles away, and my dad is tenderly showing compassion for me. My dad is telling me that he cares. This is life-changing to me.

Kid Marc shows up. Teenage Marc shows up. Young adult Marc shows up.

All the different parts of me are there to celebrate with streamers, balloons, horns! All are deeply affected in a positive way! The words of life which my dad speaks go down to my heart, and do the job of removing this unresolved block in our relationship. The impact is life-changing and I (we) will never forget it.

I have no beef at all with my dad about this anymore. It's gone.

We squared it off. It's just not there in me anymore.

I recount it mainly for the purpose of this narrative.

Forgiveness, the remission of sins, inner healing, deliverance, redemption and all the aspects of grace and the love of Jesus are wrapped around us in a big hug.

GOING FOR THE HEART

Hours later, when we make it to the summit of the Matterhorn, my dad lingers.

He holds his arms out, with a sense of achievement. He savors his triumphant arrival there with me. Something has changed within my father and he seems happier.

I think it will be even better to include my mom, especially since they made the climb together. Her presence is already imprinted in his body memory, and we will be opening up and drawing from a well deep within him. The more I include his dear Monique in our Guided Interactive Visualization Exercise, the more he will feel involved with her, and his heart will lead him closer to her...

"Look! Mom is right next to you. She's landing on that rock right next to you." My mom actually preceded my dad to the summit in reality. So I have a choice of endings, Mom arriving before or after. "Look Mom is right there, on that rock. You landed right next to her. Well done!"

I see that my dad is beginning to smile as we arrive on the mountain top. What follows at this point is out of my hands now (literally) and all about my father's reaction.

What effect will our journey have upon him?

Today, my father stays in the flying position for six minutes!

He stands there, looking out the window, stretching his arms out for six minutes. I am not holding him; I am not behind him; I am no longer holding his arms or balancing them.

What is going on here? Is he believing that I am still holding his arms? What is the power, on this day, that gives him the strength and the desire to keep these wings soaring high in the air? Is he in touch with his heart? Is he flying above the other summits that surround the Matterhorn, free in his soul like a bird?

Is he flying with his heart?

He is in another world, not a rambling or vacant world, but in a place of wonder that gives him a passion to live. Have we succeeded in creating an independent space amidst the stronghold of his disease?

I think back to our goals for him. The goals in the nonviolent struggle for democracy and living out of his heart are being achieved by the following means:

1. "By progressively growing a 'democratic space,' realized by methodically building an independent society outside of the dictatorship's control."

2. "By the use of 'nonviolent coercion.' Although the opponent's leaders remain in their positions and keep faith with their original goals, their ability to act is effectively being taken away from them." (1 and 2: Sharp, Gene. *From Dictatorship to Democracy*. The Albert Einstein Institution, 2002.)

3. The third goal reached in agreement with kid Marc: "To have him living *affectively* from the springs of life in his heart/ rather than to have him dying *effectively* from the shutting down of the life in his brain."

I will tell you that we are now moving into a new place for my dad. Helen Keller said, "One can only see rightly from the heart." She is talking about the power of love. She was blind and yet she is talking about seeing. My dad's brain is blind, yet he is expressing something that he is seeing. I love what we are doing, and it seems that my Dad loves it too.

That's when I hear back from Kid Marc.

"Dad is expressing an amazing connection to life that makes him feel good!" he says.

"Yeah!" I answer.

"And with a passion that sustains his arms up in the air for 360 seconds."

"He forgets where he is, he forgets his condition," I say seriously.

"Forgets! That's a good one!" says kid Marc laughing. "Especially since Dad feels connected again! We're not even focused on his sickness!"

"Yes it's great!" I say excitedly to my young friend, who reappears in my life as if he has never left.

"He has a purpose. And that purpose is his, and it makes him feel important," says kid Marc.

"And that purpose isn't coming from the dictator!" I say.

"So it's like he is taking his mind off his problems!"

"Kid Marc!" I answer back. "Good to hear from you! 'Taking his mind off his problems?' Are you trying to be funny?"

"That is my purpose," says kid Marc.

"It's Dad who has the new found purpose!" I quip.

"And it's a purpose outside of the dictatorship's control! We are not even fighting the disease on the terms of the dictatorship," he answers. "You remember? That was one of our objectives: 'To not let the outcome be decided by the means of fighting of the dictatorship.'"

"That's right! We are choosing our own means of fighting by building an independent state. This is independent all right," I answer.

"You could be doing this same exercise with Dad being a healthy eighty-year-old, and not sick," says kid Marc. "Without any reason to even think about regimes or revolutions!"

"Exactly, my young friend," I reply. "In many households across America, this could be a regular physical therapy exercise, designed to firm up his arm muscles, tighten his abs, improve his posture and brighten his day."

"We're just inviting his body and heart to join in the therapy and awaken," says kid Marc, enthusiastically.

"That's it! We are inviting his body and heart to awaken to the deepest sensory experiences and most memorable achievements latent within him," I add.

"Equivalent to the digging of a well, blasting through the earth's crust, striking oil that is now coming gushing up. Or finding the entrance to underground rivers of living water, unstopped and flowing through secret chambers, deep in his heart."

"Ah, the language. 'Secret chambers, deep in his heart.' I love that," I reply.

"Yeah, this is a secret chamber. His sickness loses power over him by the time he reaches the summit of the Matterhorn. He is empowered by a new strength within, and his heart soars!" says kid Marc.

"New strength from his heart. For those six minutes, I was just standing a few feet behind him," I exclaim.

"He was holding out his arms for himself! He was so caught in the moment. He loved being there. This was definitely his heart and not his head!" says kid Marc.

"He got into it, holding his arms out on the mountain. Wow. This is his heart leading him. What a break! I can't wait to see where his heart takes him," I say.

"Somewhere good, you will see. His heart will lead him to the right place," kid Marc answers me.

ROMANCE!

In view of our success, I am still thinking that I can pass on what we are doing to my mother.

This thought is again unrealistic and I have to let go of it. Like it or not, my mother's stature is shorter and her arms are in no position to assist or lead any of the exercises with my father — nor does she want to try.

However, as we continue our daily flights to the Matterhorn, my guided visualization exercise starts to play itself out in reality. Every time we land on the summit I exclaim:

"Look! There is Mom, right there, on that rock!" or:

"Mom is coming right behind us! She's coming to land, right next to you!"

After our flight ends, my mother is sitting on the white couch by the windows reading her newspaper. My father arrives — but he does not do what he always does — he does not hang out in the vicinity and stand at length by one of the side windows.

This time, he behaves totally unpredictably and walks right up to the couch. Smiling at my mom, my father makes it known that he wants to sit down on the couch next to her, and as soon as he lands, he launches into a 'conversation.'

"Cherie, I was thinking," he begins.

My mom receives this attention in a mixture of disbelief and surprise.

Her Bobby has taken an active interest in her feelings on certain matters.

"Now what do you think, Monique?"

He sits on that couch a long time with her, and while my mom cannot literally understand what he is saying, I can tell that it does not matter at all. He is pouring out his heart to her, and she enjoys that language.

She has to make room for him in her heart and in her agenda. She lets go of her newspaper, folds it and lays it down. More and more my mother opens up to receive this grace from my father, and from the Lord.

It's been years since he gave her such personal comfort, with his time, his abundance of words and his undivided attention. And he is taking the lead, and being the gentleman, crooning and courting her.

My father is now speaking the language of love.

Kid Marc is there to meet me as soon as I am back in my room.

"That was the longest time I have ever seen Dad talk with Mom on the couch in my whole life!" he exclaims.

"Unbelievable! That was way off the charts," I say.

"Do you believe it?" he says.

"Did you *see* that?" I say.

"Was that for real?" he says.

"What happened?" I say.

"He just kept talking!" he says.

"He was all lit up!" I say.

"Was that Dad on that couch?" he asks.

"Did you see Mom's face?" I exclaim.

"Dad put his arm around her!" he says.

"She was all lit up!" I say.

"Did you *see* that?" he says. And we just go round like that for a while, until we realize we keep saying the same thing.

"I am blown away," I say.

"Yeah, me too," says kid Marc.

"All this makes up for that time when I felt I wasn't being helpful. It felt like I was fixing a part of my childhood, where I could be helpful to them and make a difference," I say.

"Maybe that's why we feel so good!" says kid Marc.

All we can say in the end is: "Wow!" and "Wow! Thank you, Jesus!"

After the conversation on the couch, my father wants to spend even more time with my mom. This is great, and a huge tribute to his new found ability to live out of his heart.

The manifestation of his desire becomes most apparent around suppertime.

On a regular basis, come night time, my dad now wants to hang out in the kitchen. He comes in and sets up shop by leaning up against the stove, speaking confidently while adding animated gestures to his new found eloquence.

In his mind, he has my mom, who is stuck in the kitchen cooking dinner, all to himself. My dad, newly enjoying the attention of his Monique, flaunts like a peacock. Though my mom is preparing dinner, which is taking 90 percent of her concentration, she is also enjoying my father's company, although it seems she is also concerned about my father being too close to the stove.

He always stands in the same place, hugging the right of the stove, chatting away in words that express interest, but are hard to decipher without the skills of non-literal interpretation. My mom's non-verbal responses, spoken over the sounds and sizzle of her cooking, are perfectly pleasing to my father.

Actually, her acknowledgment of his presence only seems to encourage my dad to redouble his oratory expressions. I find it hilarious and nerve-wracking at the same time, as he reaches out his hand over the red hot stove to make a point.

My mom's quick response is: "That's hot, Bobby! You're going to burn yourself!"

My response is more direct: "Don't touch the stove, Dad!"

My father has a knack every night of misjudging the distance between his head and the metal hood over the stove.

"Oh, Bobby, you hit your head!"

My dad writes it off with a shrug that means: *This is nothing! It's just my head. You should see some of the stuff I've been through.*

For years my parents laughed at the Monty Python and Faulty Towers type of humor — a carryover from the five years my brother and I spent at a British boarding school.

My mom also loved Inspecteur Clouseau of *The Pink Panther*. So to watch my parents interact during this time of kitchen romance, where neither the heat is lacking nor the courtship, brings me right back to those situations conducted with a hysterical mixture of seriousness and buffoonery. "It's only a flesh wound," from *Monty Python and the Holy Grail,* comes to mind.

Due to the remarkable developments taking place before me each night, the humor that I am privy to, during this budding courtship unfolding before my eyes, only adds a sense of joy to the occasion. It seems that the power of suggestion influencing my Dad's behavior is bringing out the best in him, since he now fancies himself a dashing young man again, in love with his girl — who only has eyes for him.

REUNITED AT LAST

Our daily routine is now improving considerably.
It seems a cog in my father is back in place once again and he is making progress. I still rigorously maintain our shaving and identity building morning scripture time around 10:30 am, followed by the subsequent putting on of elegant clothes.

Once we are well on our way with our daily Guided Interactive Visualization Exercise, I decide to add limbering-up movements that will stretch his arms and legs.

So, before our flight over the lake and above the forest to the top of the Matterhorn, we practice arm swings. My father and I stand facing each other at arm's length. He is alert and he is paying attention.

"Okay Dad, let's swing your arms down," I say, holding his hands in mine.

I hold his hands, raise them up high, pause and let them go with a push.

My father stands there fully enjoying his arms going into motion as I send them off swinging.

Sure enough, they make their way back to me and I catch them! I hold his hands in mine, raise them high, pause and say, "Up... And down!" and send them off again.

Swinging and then waiting for the connection builds trust and creates joy. "Up! And down!"

Joy is the GREATEST healer. We could be kids swinging on a swing set, having fun. Just what kid Marc recommended to reach his heart, "Have fun with him."

"And down! And up!"

Every time I catch his hands in mine, and let them go with a push, my dad's arms come swinging back up. It is amazing to see them go flying through the air until the moment I catch them. "And up! And down!"

We can do these arm swings ten times in a row with ease. Of all the interactions I have with my father, this is the one that I enjoy the most.

Next, I set my sights on the beam across the ceiling to the left of our Matterhorn area.

I actually succeed in having my father raise his arms and place his hands on the beam above his head and then...stand on his toes.

"Dad. Now stand up on your toes!"

My naïve belief at the outset of this new stretch is: *The more enthusiastic my command, the more his heels will lift.* But Dad is not an elephant nor am I a circus trainer.

What actually is needed is another extension which tests the limits of my comfort zone. Am I willing to go beyond and extend myself physically? I am always tempted to not do it — as I have to throw my back into it, as they say, and get down on my hands and knees and push my fingers under the soles of his old blue leather slippers. It is from that lowly vantage point that I prompt him to get on his toes — with my fingers under his heels pushing them up.

There are times when all my efforts avail no results. No spark, no connection — just my fingers getting mashed between the carpet and my dad's blue leathered heels. But what keeps me going, hoping and trying, are the times when it DOES HAPPEN. When my dad stands on his toes, he breaks the mold. These victories make the effort worthwhile. To me, he overcomes every death hold by creating a neurological pathway of healing that crosses right through the enemy territory with a shout of victory: "Surprise!"

After we are done and we sit down, I often ask my dad to say his own name. "What is your name?" I say to my dad.

I cannot get him to say his own name. He knows my name and will sometimes say it: "Marc."

But when it comes to his name, I am met with a blank stare or a rambling revelation that seems to reflect a genius answer, which he is proud of. This then occasions him nodding and smiling, as if to say: "See, huh, am I good or what?" Nevertheless, genius or not, the buzzer is going off in my mind. He isn't saying his name.

One afternoon, I have a great breakthrough. I know my dad loved speaking Spanish. As a management consultant, often travelling to Spain for business, he had learned to love the Spanish people and the Spanish language.

So, I catch him by surprise. I am on the couch. He is sitting on his leather chair. I hold his eyes and say,

"Como se llamo?"

Immediately, the answer comes back:

"Me llamo Roberto."

He says it with confidence. He says his name in Spanish as if he is back in Spain, talking with a trusted friend.

My dad says his name.

As with many of the 'answers' that come to me, I have this idea when I am not thinking about it. This is the work of the Holy Spirit who is walking with me very closely, because I am committed to finding a way.

The wonderful Heavenly Comforter is our Guide and Helper. The Holy Spirit is called the "paraclete" in Greek, the one who walks along beside you. The Greek word "paralambanos" means to receive from beside you. The realm of the Holy Spirit is a rich one indeed. The word "power" or "dunamis" is ascribed to Christ — His power as King — and to the Holy Spirit's power to raise Jesus Christ from the dead, and to do mighty works of healing.

In what can feel like a maze of Alzheimer's, receiving the baptism of the Holy Spirit and being able to pray in tongues will make all the difference. "Now glory be to God, who by his mighty power at work within us is able to do far more than we would ever dare to ask or even dream of — infinitely beyond our highest prayers, desires, thoughts, or hopes. May he be given glory forever and ever..." (Ephesians 3: 20-21 TLB)

When your commitment to help your loved one is — "so close, it's scary" — the Holy Spirit will be *even closer* and be *even more* committed than you are, making order amidst chaos for you. The Holy Spirit will lead you in the same way that the jaguar is led along his or her path through the jungle — finding order in the chaos, finding light in the darkness, finding a path of grace out of the strongholds.

Don't limit your view of the Holy Spirit to the masculine only. Is not the Wisdom of God feminine in the book of Proverbs? "Happy is the man who finds wisdom, and the man who gains understanding. For *her* proceeds are better than the profits of silver, and her gain than fine gold. *She* is more precious than rubies, and all the things you may desire cannot compare with her. Length of days is in her right hand, in her left hand are riches and honor...She is a tree of life to those who take hold of her, and happy are all who retain her." (Proverbs 3:13-18 NKJ)

My lesson from the wonderful Holy Spirit along this journey is to sidestep, outwit, and circumvent the brain, and go for the heart. Get creative. Find the secret passage, the hidden tunnel, the magic garden, the open window to the heart. It's a cliché, maybe, but for a reason, because the 'wonder and awe' connection is God's path so a man doesn't get stuck in his intellect, and does find the essence of his human heart.

What is it that the heroes say in the face of their insurmountable obstacles?

"Take heart."

"Have courage."

"Just believe."

"Trust."

This takes us right back to where we started in the bathroom with my dad. "Trust in the Lord with all your heart, and lean not on your own understanding."

The heart has the power to go where the brain cannot.

Why? Because even when the brain is blind, the heart can see. The heart can trust. The heart can love.

"Reach the love in the heart and the heart will reach out in love."

Kid Marc and I coined that phrase after long weeks of being convinced that we needed to find a 'connection' with the heart.

That evening, my father is standing in the doorway of his bedroom as my mom and I are saying good night. I am not sure if he needs to go to the bathroom. I go into my room to put my water glass on the night table, joyfully thinking about the recent developments. Then I go back to look through the door that stands ajar to my mother and father's bedroom.

"Dad, do you have to go to the bathroom?"

Pause, reflection, a slight nod of his head.

The answer comes back: "Yes, I do." This is amazing to me. We have established the communication bridge. My question is in a 'yes' or 'no' format, and now he is capable of giving me a "yes" answer.

We are off to the bathroom and sure enough, he has to go. No resistance or sidetracks. I believe one day he even walked into the bathroom, and stood there in front of the bowl, taking care of business all on his own like he had been doing it all along. There is no funny talk afterward. We just walk out of there.

Every night, as I take my dad to the bathroom before going to bed, this man, who acts so sweet and loving to my mom, often speaks to me in terms of violence.

For months he had shown himself to be such a gritty, tough guy that I asked myself if he could actually have been a crime boss.

With all his talk of "wiping those guys out," and "cutting them off," he certainly is convincing in the part, acting tough as nails, gritting his teeth and motioning his hand sideways in a single decisive dismissal to pronounce judgment and pass sentence.

I am used to this daily crime boss talk; in fact, just forty-five minutes before, in the bathroom, I said: "Dad we are not 'shoving people around' anymore and 'getting rid of them.' Those days are all over." That's what I always say to him: "Those days are all over."

I say it again as I walk him by the hand into his bedroom. You know what he says back to me?

"It's just a joke!"

This is such a novel approach to his usually seriously stated consciousness of "Oh" or to the 'Who me?' enlargement of his eyes.

I am aghast.

My reaction is just as over the top a response as his: "Just a joke? Where do you get that kind of sense of humor? From the Mafia?"

He's got my mom laughing now and my dad says it again. "Yeah, it's a joke! That's great!"

Then my mom says, "It's a joke! Isn't that just about the funniest thing you've ever heard!?"

I'm laughing at my own joke which seems to have passed unnoticed. Or, to be technically correct, unheard.

I think it is pretty funny, but then my mom isn't aware of all the crime boss talk my dad has been making, which has led me to believe my dad possibly has a shady past.

I think of the Bob Dylan song, *All Along the Watchtower*, and the line: "There are some here among us who think that life is but a joke." So my mom and dad are having a wonderful time.

It's time to put Dad in his pajamas. The challenge is always whether to take off his shirt first or his pants. Mom makes the big move and gets his shirt off. She leaves his T-shirt on and we proceed to put his arms in the sleeves of the pajama top. Dad does some of the buttons, we help with the others.

Then Dad proceeds to tuck in his pajama top into his pants. I knew this was going to happen — 'dreaded' — is a better word. We are naïvely thinking that we can simply take his pants off next, but Dad is holding onto them for dear life as they are now holding his shirt in place.

Fortunately, we are still in a state of lingering laughter and my mom says:

"Bobby, you can let go of your pants now. Oh, that is just so funny!"

Dad needs to sit down to put on his pajama pants. The best place for him to do this is right where he gets into bed. We walk him around the bed and with the help of this unexpected comic interlude, pull his pants all the way down to his ankles and tell Dad to sit down on the edge of the bed.

By then Dad is quite content and Mom is saying in French: "C'est vraiment drole, tu sais!" And, as if this statement will do better in English, she says: "That was really funny, you know!"

I still think my joke is funnier, but in this emotional semi-desert, I have learned to walk humbly by myself, with an invisible Jesus at my side. So I am simply glad for the positive distraction my mother is creating, as it makes it much easier than usual to get Dad in his pajama pants. Because now he is ready to get in his bed. He is happy in bed and it is such a sense of accomplishment for all of us.

"Now just lift up your legs and you are going to be able to lie down on the bed. There you go! Very good," my mom says as she pulls up the covers to right below his chin.

"Well done, Bear! Mon ours." ("My bear," in French.)

Dad is aligned with his pillow and my mom pulls up the covers.

"There we go," my mom says. "I have the covers just like you like them. Right beneath your chin."

My father snuggles up to the covers under his chin, lights up and exclaims with a happy laugh: "A bear could catch some fish!"

Our level of relating continues to improve. He reconnects with my mom, with me, with himself and with the Lord.

In the last two weeks before he goes to the hospital my father is interacting with my mom and me.

By now we have been making our flights to the Matterhorn almost every day for three months. I incorporated a certain number of stretching exercises, but I'd never picked up the football which is sitting on the table by the stereo and tried to pass it to him.

I sent him this particular football from Tulsa as a gift because he used to love football, and I thought he would enjoy holding a football again. There has been no interest in holding much of anything since I came to Florida, but now the rules are changed.

So here we are standing in our Matterhorn area and I say: "Dad! Catch!"

I give him about three seconds to get it together before I let the ball loose, medium strength with an underhand throw. He is standing facing me, about six feet away.

You know what? I watch the ball go sailing toward him, sailing, sailing and yes, he catches it! He takes a hold of that ball with both hands and pulls it into his chest. His face shows a mixture of concentration and contentment when he catches the ball, like he has won a prize.

"Very good Dad! Good catch," I say. Then I clap my hands.

"Okay, now throw it back to me." Any attempt to try this in the past would have set the stage for any number of distractions, ending with the ball being put down somewhere as an afterthought. So even though I am used to his sidetracks, I expect him to pass the football right back to me.

After catching the ball, he lifts up his arm and throws an underhand pass right back at me, and right into my arms.

"Great throw, Dad!"

This feels great, I am actually enjoying myself. I am smiling, and thinking: *To catch the ball from my dad! My dad just threw me a football. Thank you, Lord. Amazing.*

Then he smiles, and he laughs.

I savor each pass, each moment of our five or six passes together, and I keep affirming and encouraging my dad. I want him to feel real success and a sense of achievement, so I stop while we are ahead.

"Good catch!"

My father never drops the ball or drifts off during our passing exchange.

One hundred percent success.

"That is great Dad!" I say as he is squarely throwing me back the football for the last time. "You did great! Well done. I really enjoyed that."

Later on that evening, my father connects with my mom in the most beautiful way. My mother is putting her Bob to bed. The nightstand light is on and there is a soft glow around them.

My dad is lying with his head on the pillow under the covers looking very content. He is smiling up at my mother, a big happy smile and she is beaming back at him. Then they start to laugh. They keep looking at each other with love eyes, and keep laughing.

The scene is so tender and touching that I want to get my camera, but the light is too low.

'It doesn't matter,' I think. 'It's okay. I will never forget this.'

One camera shot will never capture all the treasured love before me, and I am glad that I didn't miss out on *living* the moment by leaving them to go get my camera.

Life, when it happens, is a precious gift to be T-R-E-A-S-U-R-E-D in a world of mostly missed connections. Even one such instance is enough to savor for a lifetime in the heart of a grateful soul. There are no guarantees. This might be the only one, or the beginning of more, and the thought that it is setting a precedent is cause for great rejoicing in heaven and on earth.

I live the moment and I capture it by living it. That night my sore body and watchful heart can let go and breathe out.

Thank God, I think. *Thank you, Lord of love and grace.*

DAD FALLS

The next day after dinner, my dad suddenly loses all the strength in his legs.

Once he stands up from the dining room table he can only walk a few steps. Both my mom and I are there. I am holding his hand and trying to hold him on his feet and keep him from falling.

"Get the chair over here," I call out to my mom. She puts the chair against the wall right behind him and I steer him down into it. My dad has always been able to walk, very slowly most of the time, but always able to walk.

This is a major problem and it comes as a complete surprise. The immediate issue is that he cannot spend the night on that chair, which places a lot of stress on me since I am going to have to somehow carry him down the hallway and onto his bed.

I think about the best way to do this and I remember from rock climbing that the longer we wait, the harder it will be. He will only get heavier and harder to move and less cooperative.

My mom is aware of the present difficulty and looks to me for the next step. I tell her my plan and begin the laborious task of lifting my father's arms over my shoulders and slowly pulling him behind me.

I am already taxed and this effort of carrying my father down the hallway is absolutely exhausting. His sheer weight squeezes out most of my strength before I am even halfway down the hallway.

My mother puts a chair in the hallway and I sit Dad down in it and take a break.

My mom is saying: "Oh Bobby, what happened to you?"

"He is going to be OK, Mom," I say. "Please help me Lord," I pray, then I once again lift my dad's arms over my shoulders and drag him behind me. The remainder of the journey is extremely difficult.

I am on my own to carry him, and it is evident how much I have carried him on my own all these previous months. I feel like I am carrying a much incapacitated man. His body has gone limp, and he is utterly unable to use his muscles in any way. By a miracle, I drag him into the bedroom to his bed and somehow lay him down on the sheet with his head on the pillow. My mom pulls up the blanket close to his chin. She is afraid, yet grateful that Bob is finally in bed after this long ordeal. I go to bed exhausted and immediately fall asleep.

In the wee hours of the morning, I wake up, jarred out of a deep sleep with the sound of my mother crying out: "Oh no, Bobby!"

What is going on? I get up, walk into the hallway and slowly open the door to my parent's bedroom, which was left ajar the night before.

The bed sheets and blankets are pulled to the side and my father has ended up on the floor, without any clothes on, naked and leaning back against his night table. 'Slouching' would be a better word. Can it get any worse? By the horrified look on my mother's face, I can tell there is more and I approach my father to see him closer.

He is covered in diarrhea everywhere. 'Everywhere' meaning even between his toes, under his nails and behind his ears. I am already exhausted from having to carry him to the bedroom the night before, with him leaning his whole weight on me and walking at a snail's pace from the dining room down the hallway to the bedroom. Physically it is the hardest thing I've ever had to do. I'm sure that months and months of taking care of him have taken its toll on my physical strength.

Nevertheless, the situation is not acceptable. Mom and I undertake the humbling task of cleaning him up — working as a team — going back and forth with hot washcloths and wiping him clean everywhere, including under his toenails and under his fingernails. Then we clean up the carpet around him.

Following our clean-up, my father is still slouched and he seems — unable to move. Due to the extent of my exhaustion, I feel that I am in no way ready to pick him up again.

"Can you try?" my mom asks me.

I brace myself and take hold of my dad's arms and lean back to pull him up. He starts to get up off the floor but soon crumples under the weight of his own body.

"What shall we do?" my mom asks.

"Even if I get him on the bed, then what? I still can't move him anywhere else," I say to my mom. "Whatever we decide to do, we are going to need to get him around. Why don't I find a medical store and go get Dad a wheelchair?"

"That is a very good idea, Marc."

So off I go towards Altamont in my parent's Bonneville, that I have polished and waxed a couple of times on previous visits, to keep it looking good. I feel the Lord is with me. I am praying and thinking, *Mom didn't even think of calling 911 at any point. I am glad she didn't.*

I do not want to have two men my father does not know come in an emergency vehicle and find him naked and lying on the floor after all the dignity and honor I have been trying to restore to him.

This morning, I am caring for my dad in person.

On a deeper level it is hard to let go, and hard to admit that my father might be needing to go to the hospital, and that this is the beginning of him never coming back home again.

I certainly am not focused on that. In fact, deep down I have great peace. I also have a sense of urgency, which I communicate to the lady at the medical supply store when I get there.

"We close in half an hour, so it is good that you called us ahead of time," she says. "Sometimes we leave early on Saturday mornings."

She helps me choose a wheelchair.

At the counter, about to check out, I start spilling out all the events of the morning. I have seen so many doors open and miracles happen simply because I open up my mouth and share my current situation.

"My dad is not standing on his own and he is going to need a wheelchair for me to move him. He ended up lying on the floor beside his bed this morning, naked and covered in his own poop."

"Oh, diarrhea is a sign of dehydration," she says. "That can cause some serious conditions. That can be very bad for him. I would take him to the hospital as soon as possible."

I stand before this lady in awe and very grateful.

"Oh, dehydration, sure. Yeah, I need to get him to the hospital. Thank you, you saved my life, or my dad's life anyway!"

"Yeah, get him there today. Hope it goes well. All my best to you and your father!"

THE GLORY OF GOD

By now the staff has gathered at the front. Helping people medically is what they do, and to be able to help makes everyone feel fulfilled. They walk me to the door and help put the wheelchair in the large trunk of this champagne-colored Bonneville. I see them starting to close up the store as I am leaving.

Well, that changed my life! I start thinking. "Wow, Lord, thanks for being there for me. Thank you! Wow, that was close!"

It was close. It is one of those defining moments in this story. I feel good, and I have a sense of gratitude for my new support team. My first reaction is to pray. "Do I call 911? Do I call my mom?" Calling 911 is not what I feel led to do. I call my mom. No answer. *Yes, it is better to tell my mom face to face. I am only a half hour away from the apartment,* I think.

"Help me, Lord. Help me tell my mom. Help me move my dad."

It is a glorious day and all around me I feel a great love and that my Father God is very pleased with me. I allow myself to let go and be in the moment on the drive 'home.'

I roll down the windows and feel the breeze and take in the sights of the palm trees and the big puffy clouds. The Florida clouds are as beautiful as if I am flying way up high in the air, 'cruising at an altitude of 30,000 feet,' as the American Airlines captain says, and looking at the world from above the clouds.

I come home and push the wheelchair onto the elevator. Getting out on the fifth floor, I stop to look at the beautiful view. I cast my cares on the Lord.

I need a word from the Lord. He speaks to me very kindly: "Fear not. Have courage. I am with you. As long as you get him there sometime tonight, he will be OK."

Jesus says: "Fear not. For I am with you," (which is found in Isaiah 43: 1-5), and I am encouraged. He gives me His peace. He will work everything out. I roll the wheelchair down the balcony to apartment 515 and go in.

I tell Mom that Dad is dehydrated and that we have to take him to the hospital this evening. She receives the report with some trepidation. "If we could take him to the hospital ourselves, I would prefer that," she says. "To have an ambulance coming in here, all sirens blaring, in front of all the neighbors, I just don't want to do that. Please think of how disorienting to Dad that would be, to have them put him on a stretcher, strap him up, he is not dressed..."

"I agree Mom. Let's give him the dignity of getting him ready ourselves."

"Thank you, Marc."

"Mom, what about confirming this with Dad's doctor?"

"It is Saturday. Very hard to reach him. Besides, I am sure that was the Lord speaking to us in the lady from the medical store."

"I feel like as long as we get him in tonight, he will be all right."

My mom sets out to take care of some personal matters while I am left facing my dad, who is still naked and slouching on the floor.

I line up the wheelchair behind me and look up to pray: "Lord, please, you've got to help me now. I really need your help."

Now is the time to get my father off the floor. We need to get him dressed. I tried hours earlier to get him on his feet, but he was too weak to get up. Like he had done the night before, he went limp and immediately crumpled and dropped back down under the weight of his own body.

This time, I feel differently. My father has to get up; we must go to the hospital. My mom is back and standing next to me, all prepared, with his pants and belt, tee shirt and shirt.

She is looking alternately at me, then at my dad now all cleaned up, with the carpet around him cleaned up, but still naked on the carpet, and still leaning back against his night table.

"Do you think you can get him up?" my mom says to me.

"Yes, he's going to get up."

There are no options; he has to get on his feet. My plan is based on the healing of "the man lame from birth," in Acts 3: 1-9:

> "There was a lame man sitting at the gate called "Beautiful." As Peter and John were passing by, he asked them for some money. They looked at him intently, and then Peter said, "Look here!" The lame man looked at them eagerly, expecting a gift. But Peter said, "We don't have any money for you! But I'll give you something else! I command you in the name of Jesus Christ of Nazareth, walk!" Then Peter took the lame man by the hand and pulled him to his feet. And as he did, the man's feet and ankle-bones were healed and strengthened so that he came up with a leap, stood there for a moment and began walking! Then, walking, leaping, and praising God, he went into the temple with them. When the people inside saw him walking and heard him praising God, and realized he was the lame beggar they had seen so often at The Beautiful Gate, they were inexpressibly surprised! They all rushed out to Solomon's Hall, where he was holding tightly to Peter and John! Everyone stood there awed by the wonderful thing that had happened." (NKJ).

I look at my father and say: "Dad, Jesus loves you. God values you. He gave his Son for you. You are not made to be lame on the ground but to walk like me. You are going to stand up now. Ready?"

I brace myself squarely in a position to pull him up, by holding his wrists firmly, and wedging my bare feet over the top of his bare feet. I want him to stand up right where he is, and not slip forward.

I start leaning back, pulling his arms.

Then I say the command with a loud voice: "Dad, stand up in the name of Jesus!"

My father stands right up! And, he stays standing there.

This is definitely the healing power of Jesus.

My mom is very happy. I am relieved and grateful, and by a continuing miracle he stays standing and we manage to dress him. At this point, my mom leaves to get some things ready for the hospital.

So my father is still standing there, even though my mom has moved the wheelchair right behind him, ready for him to sit in once he is dressed.

Quite suddenly a change of appearance overtakes him.

As he is standing there, he becomes full of the might of the Lord. Not like a general in warfare, more like a president, a great leader. Jesus is in him, as a great leader of government.

The Lord's presence inside of Bob is so strong; it is almost too much for my human flesh to bear. It knocks me back a step. I feel like Daniel for a moment, when he is in the presence of the Angel of God, and he says: "How can such a person as I even talk to you?" (Daniel 10: 17-20 TLB). I don't feel weak like Daniel, but I am still moved backward by the presence of the Lord in Bob.

Bob is a great man in your Kingdom and he is your son and he is clean inside. That is my thought. *Clean in his soul.*

The light of the Lord is here and the revelation of His Holy Spirit is clear.

And at this moment I know one thing for sure: the evil spirit that tried holding him in bondage his whole life has cleared out. The incest from his mother or whatever horrible name it is called — is gone.

There is no way he can be filled with the presence of the Lord to this degree and still have any evil spirits attached to him. After one last fling as the evil spirit drives Dad to smear his own diarrhea all over his body, my dad is delivered from the attachment of this evil spirit.

It is gone. It left him, then we cleaned him up and now he is dressed and in his right mind.

"Dad, you are all clean inside," I say out loud to my father. I know he cannot be so full of the Lord and so blessed with the honor and glory of His presence, unless he is clean.

My dad is looking so strong, after being so weak. He is looking so healthy after being all limp; he is looking so fit after being slouched and dehydrated for 24 hours. My father is healed and his inner man is full of the Lord and safe in His care.

I am in awe in the presence of my Dad's 'transfiguration.' I also am touched by the powerful impact of Dad's positive light-filled presence as it eases the toll that months of evil have had upon me. The load lifts from my chest.

I am glad for this miraculous boost of energy in which my father becomes a man restored to his dignity, holding himself with honor and strength. As we stand together facing each other, there is an impartation of that strength from him to me.

I feel his pleasure and I realize my father has imparted his blessing to me. After all we have been through I am wide open and pleased to receive the blessing of my father!

My mother is in another room, and it is just the two of us in the bedroom, as my father imparts his mantle to me and his blessing.

But wasn't he out of it, wasn't he passed the point of no return — incapable of having such power? Wasn't the devil-disease-dictatorship in charge? Not anymore at this point it seems, because there is a coup, a veritable revolution happening before my eyes, run by an independent society that can manifest supernatural strength in Bob from the same Holy Spirit who brought Jesus Christ back from the dead. The glory of the Lord in Bob is so strong, and I am a part of it, and I receive the mantle and the blessing that is mine as a gift from my father through the Lord.

Whatever will happen next, I know, all *will* be well.

Following this momentous event, it is time to walk my dad back to the wheelchair and help him sit down.

He is content and he looks out of the window, and, as the sun is shining in upon him he is smiling.

My mom returns with a sense of urgency and knows we need to leave for the hospital. It is already six, and I tell her what the Lord said to me: "As long as we are there sometime this evening, Dad will be OK." Dad is directly behind Mom, still looking out of the window and smiling. I know he will be OK. Deep down I have great peace. For I know this: before Dad went into the hospital I had an experience of him being strong and clean inside. It happened after the most difficult night and his last night ever at home.

Now he is all cleaned up, dressed, and seated in his wheelchair. We decide to take him to the hospital. We make our way out of the apartment into the beautiful tropical world of palm trees, red rooftops and Mediterranean architecture as it is seen from this fifth-floor balcony-hallway.

We are standing, waiting for the elevator, and I am looking across at the three palm trees that symbolize so much of my parent's life here. I look at my dad in the wheelchair. He is going with the flow, not resisting or chatty, but calm. He seems to be appreciating the gift of this moment and of his life here. I am very aware that this is the last time he will ever be in the presence of these three majestic palm trees, and that he is no longer coming back to this apartment.

Yet the sun is shining upon us in such a hopeful way. My mom seems anxious and I don't want her to miss this moment, but now is not the time for a life lesson on trusting God and not being anxious. As the elevator drops slowly down, floor by floor, I feel like I have lived that moment which marks the end of an era. The memory of it is in the warm feeling of sunshine on my face, and the honor and dignity in my father's composure.

Dad gets in the front seat easily, positioning his loafers comfortably on the camel-colored floor mat, almost without my help. I fold up the wheelchair and put it in the trunk. We drive to the Florida Hospital on Lakemont Avenue. As I park their Bonneville in the emergency entrance, we are met by a friendly staff member who brings out a wheelchair for my father. Dad graciously gets out of the car and we help him sit down.

We are ushered into an ICU unit fairly quickly and nurses come in to assess the situation. They conduct blood tests and a doctor comes in to talk with us, as they are putting Dad on an IV.

"Mrs. Swift, I am Dr. Rami. You did well to bring in your husband tonight. The tests confirm that he is extremely dehydrated. He also has a bladder infection. We are going to put him on intravenous fluids to hydrate him. Unfortunately, his blood stream has some infection as well."

"His blood stream is infected?" says my mom.

"There is still time to treat this problem before his organs are adversely affected. We are going to need to put a catheter on him to help with his urine flow."

Dr. Rami leaves and a nurse comes in and unwraps the plastic packaging to pull out the catheter. This, of course, is painful to watch, especially as the nurse has to ask for another nurse to help her, after an unsuccessful first attempt.

Then another, more relaxed looking doctor comes in and introduces himself.

"Hi, Mrs. Swift. Hi Marc. I am Dr. Karol. Your husband is extremely dehydrated and we are taking care of that. He will be fine. He also has a classic case of bladder infection. I see these cases a lot. I actually have a lady who comes in *regularly* with her husband when he gets a bladder infection. She always says she can tell, because he starts acting a little crazy. In Bob's case, the infection has spread to his blood stream and we want to do all we can to counteract the poison from affecting him adversely."

"Is it serious?" asks my mom.

"It would be a problem if it couldn't be treated. But Bob is here in our care now and you can go home tonight in peace. He is going to be fine."

"Thank you, Dr. Karol, for your help," we both say feeling relieved.

We walk with transport when Dad is ready to be moved to his room. It is a private room, and soon we have to leave him.

Alone for the first time.

While it is a relief to know my dad will get the treatment he needs, there is a strange emptiness in the apartment as we return.

I have to remind myself of the miracle I witnessed short hours before, as the sun was streaming through the window. My father was full of the strength of the Lord, clean inside and he gave me his blessing!

I say goodnight to my mom and go into my 'room.' I am inspired to write a poem after being face to face with the Glory of the Lord in my dad.

Let the Gates of Heaven ring out and sing,
For to the earth, did God His Glory bring!

HOW AM I SUPPOSED TO FEEL?

The next day, all is different with Dad.

He is the opposite of the glory I experienced the day before.

I am so torn up about it that I have to talk to my son Josh, and write out my feelings in my journal that night, after being with him all day.

My Journal Entry:

Josh, how am I supposed to feel about this??

My dad is stuck in the hospital; he has a tube out of his penis. He thrashes around in different levels of pain.

Even though he has teeth, he sounds like a man whose dentures are out of his mouth, rounded words that sound incapacitated.

We get excited at the glimmer of a recognizable phrase. He seems to be saying to my mom: "My sweet angel."

We have to feed him now. That was the one thing he could do on his own, to cheers of, "Dad eats so well. He eats everything on his plate, right up to the last rice kernel."

Now he is wearing mittens on his hands so he won't pull out his catheter. He is not eating much and the food hangs on his mouth, caught in his bristly skin.

How am I supposed to feel about this???
It is too close,

and more than I can bear...
warfare,
war, war, war.
Jesus has conquered death, sickness, Satan.
Won over them.
Healthy- vibrant- alive- beautiful- life- joy- expression,
Giving, thoughtful,
They are there in Jesus, but not here now;
even though I do see his strong connection to Mom, it is
still more than
I can bear...
Have mercy, Lord, help me!!!!!!!!!!
HOPE...needed,
God needed,
A cross needed,
a cross to put this on.
Jesus bore it. Jesus bore it,
became it.
Lord, help! You bore it, Jesus...
"Surely He has borne our griefs and carried our sorrows;
Yet we esteemed Him stricken, smitten by God and
afflicted.
But He was wounded for our transgressions,
He was bruised for our iniquities:
The chastisement for our peace was upon Him,
And by His stripes we are healed." (Isaiah 53:5 NKJ)

"It seems so cruel. I hate it!" rings out the reaction of my senses but deep down I do have great peace. For I know this: before Dad went into the hospital I had an experience of him being strong and clean inside.

Now, as I am feeling all these emotions, standing next to him, as he is lying on his hospital bed, my father calls me "son." It is the first time he's ever called me "son." It is the first time in my life that I can remember. To call me "son" means that he is my dad. Looking like this.

Or maybe he is hearing his heavenly Father saying that he is the 'son.' Bob, "the beloved son of the Father," which I told him he was, day after day, for months while I was shaving him.

"You are the beloved son of the Father," I would say to my dad. "Dad, the Father says to you: 'Fear not, for I am with you. Nothing will ever be able to separate you from my love.'"

My dad does get better, the pain lessens. He stays in the hospital two more weeks until we get a call at the apartment from the doctor in charge saying he will be releasing Dad the following day.

My mom protests. We are spending most of the day in the hospital. No doctor has come to talk with us about releasing dad. And my mom is not ready for my dad to just 'come home.' Her protest eventually results in another doctor taking the case load, and extending Dad's stay, and making a decision to put Dad on a medication called Seroquel.

The day comes when we have to take my father out of the hospital. My mom decides to put him in a nursing home. We come to this decision after consulting with several representatives from Winter Park nursing homes, who come by his room at the hospital at my mom's request. Bringing Dad back home is not realistic; my mom cannot handle this possibility. She is too tired.

We go to Regents Park, which at first sight seems like a friendly place for a nursing home, but turns out to be a horrible place. Dad ends up having a stroke on the third day he is there.

Of course, there the Lord always has an encouraging person in these kinds of places and that is Dad's roommate, Jim. Jim is there in the bed next to Dad, and we have a great talk with this man who is the Lord's blessing to us.

The next morning, we come back to see Dad. I spot him first, as we are making our way to his room. He is sitting in a wheelchair in the middle of the hallway.

I say to Mom: "Look, there is Dad."

"Where?" she asks.

"Right there," I say.

"That's not Dad," she says.

"Yeah, that's Dad," I say.

"That's not Dad," she says again. It is very hard for my mom to accept that she is looking at her husband.

After a long time, she says: "I wouldn't have recognized him."

Dad looks dead, void of feeling, like some great big vacuum cleaner has sucked the life out of him. I hate it.

There is some kind of evil in a place like this where somebody, somewhere is getting off on sucking men and women's souls and enjoying the power of seeing them helpless.

The devil has the illusion that he has actually succeeded in stealing these men and women's souls forever. But I am here to tell you that Jesus will have the last word. This is the Good News: All who want to be with Jesus, will be with Him.

This is the good news that Jesus went to preach to the souls in Sheol after his death on the cross — "He descended into hell and on the third day He arose from the dead" is what the Apostle's Creed says. He descended into hell and preached eternal Victory over death, sin, and Satan to all the helpless souls who seemed like they were lost forever. Then He brought them back up with Him, in His glory train right through the gates of heaven. "Lift up your heads, O you gates! And be lifted up you everlasting doors! And the King of Glory shall come in. Who is this King of Glory? The LORD strong and mighty, The LORD mighty in battle." (Psalm 24: 7-10 NKJ).

The way God's compassion extends to my mom and me in this nursing home is that I recognize from the downward curve on his mouth, that my dad has had a stroke.

I am quite sure that the stroke happened either as a result of the Seroquel or because of the over-extended, vigorous physical therapy my father received earlier that day, or both. The nursing home had a hard time accepting the fact that my father had a stroke on their watch, given the possible legal ramifications. I continue to trust the Lord for Dad and see no value in starting to level accusations against them or start legal action. I have to choose. Be angry against the nursing home or stay lovingly focused on my father. I can't do both.

It still takes two days to get the administration of the nursing home to let him go, but the ambulance comes and takes him back to the hospital — this time to the cardiac floor.

Gina, a nurse we already know, is there to greet us and take care of Dad, for which we are very grateful. I hear the patient in the bed next to Dad snoring and it seems like a dark room, but it is late. One thing that seems out of place and definitely encouraging is a Toastmaster-like timing light on the table at the nurse's station. The Green Light is on. That is pretty cool. It felt like, yeah, God wants us here. Dad is in room 3405 and my mom comments that it has a lot more class than the room on the first floor, where we were the first time.

We do not yet realize the impact of the stroke — Dad is no longer able to eat or drink — but it is a huge relief to get out of the nursing home. We celebrate the miracle of this weekend, with special thanks to the Lord for Dad surviving the nursing home and being back in the hospital.

My mom tries to stay in touch with my brother Greg by phone, to apprise him of the new developments, but he is very busy travelling on business so he never takes the time to become involved with caring for Dad. It's funny because he was always the responsible one growing up, and I was the 'screw up,' the black sheep of the family. Yet here I am being the one to help my dad, while he is gone on business or otherwise occupied.

PENTECOST SUNDAY

I t is 6:40 am.
From the moment I wake up this Sunday morning of Pentecost, I feel God very kindly beckoning me into his goodness. Sure enough, even this morning before going to the hospital, I feel the warm outpouring of his love and goodness, beckoning me to put on a multi-color shirt. *Celebrate Jesus, today,* I am thinking. "Thank you, Jesus for giving us Your Holy Spirit today!"

This morning, Pam, my neighbor in Tulsa, calls me. Tree branches have fallen down in my backyard in Tulsa and that is why she is calling me. The big branches fell in the yard and spared the house completely, and missed the fence and the power line. What a great hand of protection the Lord has over my house in Tulsa.

She said more winter nights will be forthcoming. I pray: "Lord Jesus please cover my house with your hand, and cover all of the cul-de-sac and the whole neighborhood so that no tornadoes or heavy-duty winds can do any more damage to that area. Please protect every single limb and tree, no more damage, thank you, Jesus. Amen." The Lord did continue to protect the house after that. No more branches fell and my friend Janice helped by having Carlos, my friend and tree genius, get it all cleaned up.

In the hospital room with Dad this morning, a strong nurse named Korbet gives us the complete medical rundown of all that Dad has been through and what their concerns are and what he's doing in this heart unit called Special Progressive Care Unit.

He tells us that his Troponin levels went high, which indicates that an 'event' happened. What the consequences of this event are, they are not sure, but they know for sure that an event happened. If there was a small stroke, and it affected his swallowing, they would be staying on the safe side, because he is non-responsive. That's why he is on the IV.

If needed, in two or three days they would get him a *banana bag* full of all kinds of nutrients. Was all this caused by the wrong medicine, we ask? Or the physical therapy? They are not sure. But here they can monitor his heart and he can rehabilitate. Every person's body is different. The nurse tells us that Dr. Cambridge would be coming in to examine Dad this afternoon. So we stay and order some lunch.

As we finish eating, in comes Dr. Cambridge. Both he and I are nervous because I'm very aware that I challenged him about the definition of 'dementia' in his office many months ago, and I'm thinking he probably doesn't like me. So I am asking the Lord, really fast, if he can make that go away, and establish a new relationship. Dr. Cambridge is looking at me a little distrustfully but I stay cool and I show respect for him.

He goes to check Dad out with a knee-jerk reflex and my mom asks a question, about the observation that my dad just doesn't seem to be responsive. He explains that what matters is that it has to be the same response on both sides. Then he comes over and taps my mom's knees for their knee-jerk reflex.

At that point I say to him: "All right! So that was a bonus!"

He loves it and starts laughing wholeheartedly and from then on I know that we are friends. It just gets better after that, although we hit a wall when he says, "Because of the Alzheimer's, I am going to put him on_____, an Alzheimer's medication."

My mother counters his helpful offering by saying: "But, last time you said that he was too far gone for any kind of medication.

I know my mom and she is saying: "How come you are changing your tune now?"

Dr. Cambridge winces but humbly answers: "Well it was hard to say what state he was in. Maybe he already had the bladder infection and I mistook that as his condition."

I am thinking, *I don't think so.*

He is maybe thinking *here we go with the affronts again,* but it is obvious he wants to help and be involved.

My mother misses the opportunity to talk about Dad's new connection with us. She does not mention how he's been chatting away with her in the kitchen every night, and on the couch. She does not mention his flights to the Matterhorn every day, or his throwing the football back and forth with me. My mom also declines to ask him what his diagnosis would be of Bob's Alzheimer's condition today, for him to be offering medication to my father at this point. My mother has been dominating the conversation with Dr. Cambridge, leaving me no open space to pitch in. No invitation to talk about the power of freeing his body memory, or of reaching his heart. When she drops the subject I am not happy, though the doctor is relieved to not have to face a confrontation. He looks happy.

I am totally not satisfied with Dr. Cambridge's answer: "Maybe, he already had the bladder infection." I know that a lot has happened to explain my father's change in condition today.

I am making a face and kid Marc shows up. He says: "But why is he saying the medication can help now?"

"Exactly! I thought Dad was too far gone!"

"You want to know?" says kid Marc.

"Yes," I say.

"In a word, because there is improvement," kid Marc replies.

"Improvement. Yes! Amen!" I say. "Thank you for helping me see all the improvement we have made, kid Marc."

Improvement.

It is true. What about all our times of shaving in the bathroom? Each day of the week repeating the same scriptures to him. He received God's words to him and even said them with me. "Trust in the Lord with all your heart."

I add up the numbers. I gave Dad 300-500 'non-literal interpretations' to his comments, during the five months from November 22, 2012, to April 27, 2013. Together with Dad, we did the Guided Interactive Visualization Exercise flights to the Matterhorn every day for an average of six days a week (a total time of almost 2000 minutes). Plus, there was my constant caring presence, and my faith — combined with my mother's faith and her sharing the load, especially of his bathroom needs at night.

Improvement. Yes, after casting out the evil spirits of defiance and mockery three times a day for two months, there was improvement. After putting him in line over and over, affirming the positive, and disciplining, correcting, and rebuking his mean comments to me, as strongly and creatively as I could, there is improvement.

The day he went to the hospital he was delivered from the stronghold spirit that had held him captive all his life — the spirit of lust and incest from his mother. I witnessed this deliverance with my own eyes. I saw my father afterward, full of honor and dignity. He was clean inside his soul and at peace with God, at peace with us and at peace with himself. And the most important of all this to me: he was ready to enter eternal life.

That's Improvement, which came as the result of working things through, setting things right, getting ready for the big one, the party of a lifetime — being welcomed with open arms into the everlasting Kingdom of our Lord and Savior Jesus Christ. That is a good place to be for any man.

Dr. Cambridge now leaves with a thumbs-up gesture, then surprises us both by coming back after half an hour to tell us: "No wonder he is in such bad shape, between the bladder infection, the dehydration, and the Seroquel medication." He says: "All that would do anybody in." He is definitely happy.

He says there will be no permanent damage from the medication and Bob will be in much better shape once they take care of these problems. So we laugh some more and he leaves with a big smile and a very kind look to me.

It is very kind of him. Not sure how everything will work out for Dad, but he has been keeping a smile on his face, and is at peace. Not sure how everything will work out for Dad, but he has been keeping a smile on his face, and is at peace.

NO FOOD OR THE PEG?

Dr. Varnedore, the neurologist, comes in to tell us about our options. During the almost 45-minute talk, we are standing by Dad's bed. We have to make a decision. Where do we draw the line? He can't drink or eat anymore.

She says: "If he was one of my family members, I would put a peg in his stomach." She would not let the person starve to death. Basically, what she is saying is that: "when someone is in this kind of condition, it tends to get worse if he's not eating."

She also says that a family member of hers was in Vitas Hospice, which is very nearby, and it was a really good experience. Another thing to consider, she says, is that without my Dad being able to respond to commands, they will not be able to do any physical therapy.

Michelle comes in to see us with a concerned look on her face after Dr. Varnadore leaves. She says that she can call Hospice to ask someone to come tomorrow to talk to us. Yes, we agree, and she arranges for the nurse from Hospice to meet us at 10 am.

The very long day comes to a close and we go for dinner at Brio. There we meet Tom, our waiter, a friendly young man studying to become an English teacher. He could have been my son Josh. We kick it off, talking about English and I tell him about my book, and we have a very spirited, enthusiastic conversation. I am going to have to find a way to meet this young man again and talk with him some more, I tell myself.

During our dinner at Brio's, Mom and I talk about Dr. Varnadore's recommendation to have a surgeon put a 'peg' in Dad's stomach to 'feed' him. I'm not sure how we've come to even consider this option. Does being in this fancy restaurant, surrounded by such ease and luxury, enhance our discernment process? I doubt it. I feel a bit dulled, even as I am asking the Lord to help us.

Honestly, coming here is my mother's idea and the way she is dealing with my dad's condition. My mother loves Brio's and she is finding comfort here. It is a place where she and Dad have come many times in the past 20 years. This vivacious restaurant filled with European charm holds many good memories for her.

I'm not sure this has much to do with reality, though. If I passed around pictures of my dad in his hospital bed would I get a lot of 'oohs' and 'aahs?' For my part, I am hungry and glad to eat. I am also very aware of the contrast, my dad not being able to eat while we are being offered a variety of delicacies, soups, salads and desserts on top of the big main entrées.

The good thing is that I am with my mom and she is not having to go through this alone. That is something to celebrate.

We manage to get a good sleep that night and arrive a little after 10am, to Dad's room, number 3405. Sandra is there and we pull up three chairs from behind the nurses' station and sit together in the hallway. Talking with Sandra is humbling but wonderful as we soon realize we are still responding at a very superficial level.

There is a lot more involved with both bringing Dad home — and, most of all, with putting a peg in his stomach. By the time we are done, there are so many reasons not to put in the peg. Thank God He sent Sandra to stop the procedure.

Somehow my mother said "Yes" to the surgery the day before, and they were setting up to do it. Here the Lord steps in very gently and opens our eyes.

Just like Him.

So we realize, for ourselves, that it's like using a manual machine in Dad's stomach; it feeds him — but it's not natural; someone has to be there always, always, always, to feed him, to get the amounts right and it's totally liquid — and that often creates a lot of diarrhea.

Been there, done that! is what both my mom and I are thinking. We are convinced. Besides it is 'extraordinary means,' an unnatural way of prolonging Dad's life and he would never want that. Neither do we, after talking with Sandra.

"Thank you, Sandra. Yes, this is clearly not the way to go for Bob," my mom says to Sandra. "Thank God we met with you this morning."

Sandra answers: "Yes, I cannot tell you the number of people I have talked to who have said to me, 'We wish we had never done this!'"

"Can you help us?" my mom says.

"I have an open bed available in Hospice today for Bob if you would like to have it."

She has an open bed available in Hospice. Today. For Dad, I am thinking. *It is a small ward. It could get filled up tomorrow. Wow, this is a very special opening. Sure seems like an invitation from You, Lord. Thank you, Jesus.*

"Okay, let me pray about this for a minute," my mom says to Sandra.

My mom tells me she hears the Lord say, "He needs to go there today. No peg, no tube."

I feel the same way and support her decision.

"Mom, it's an open door," I say. "There is a bed ready. This is the day. Time for Dad to go to Hospice. Thank you, Jesus for Your grace."

Mom returns to Sandra. "Yes, Sandra, please bring Bob to Hospice," my mother says.

Sandra smiles, "I will let everyone know."

After we decide to transfer Dad to Hospice, the whole team comes into the hospital room at lunch time: Linda, Dad's nurse,

185

along with Grace, then Dr. Varnedore and Dr. Shah, followed by Dr. Reddy. They stand around Robert Swift's bed in a circle, almost as if they are going to hold hands, knowing what we decided about not using the peg and transferring him to Hospice.

It is a sacred moment. The unseen presence of the Lord fills the space between us. We all stand around Dad's bed as if gathered before the counsel fire of the elders. They give us their approval and best wishes and hopes to support our decision not to intervene by using "extraordinary means" to "save, prolong, fix, or sustain" Dad.

I speak up now, addressing our doctors and nurses, as we gather around Dad's bed, "My friends, thank you for all your loving care for my dad. You have gone over and above in your dedication to help him, for which we are very grateful. I think we can all agree, that if God wants to do a miracle with my dad, He can do it and He doesn't need a peg to do it. He can fix his throat, get him drinking again and eating again. God doesn't need our intervention by extraordinary means to do it. We are not going to take this matter into our own hands, but trust in the Lord."

My speech results in nods of affirmation, some "um-hums," and finally someone says, "That's right!" We are in agreement. Everyone leaves.

Dr. Reddy comes back to tell us Hospice will come and get Dad tomorrow evening, Memorial Day, Monday, at 6pm. Dr. Shah comes and tells us she will be back tomorrow to check him out, and make sure all is well, before the transfer to Hospice.

EHE—DENA—CHI

After this long day, we are very hungry and it is time to go out and eat. My mom wants to go across the street to Outback for dinner. I am hungry, but I don't feel that I can enjoy a big meal.

We arrive home and I am weighed down by the finality of our decision. I am tired and go to sleep, but then I arise in the middle of the night and violently jump out of bed. I keep saying: "My father can't die without being able to drink any more water!!"

A sudden panic seizes me. I keep saying, "My father is never going to drink water again?! He has to be able to drink water again! It is time for Dad to drink water again, Jesus. Please Jesus!"

The realization comes so forcefully to me that I pace almost frantically in circles, being in torment at the thought of Dad never having any more water, waving my arms in disbelief, and shouting "No!" almost to the point of exhaustion, until a peace comes over me, in the form of a thought:

I will find a way! My father will have water to drink.

I make my peace by declaring that I will find a way to hydrate him every day. I resolve to find a way to keep water in his mouth, even if it is only a little water every day. Yes, if I keep giving him a little, it will be enough. It can be absorbed into his system, and maybe he can even swallow a small amount.

Memorial Day, Monday

Dad is lying in bed in this cardiac care room, and he is quiet. Mom and I are facing the door, which is open to the hallway where there are doctors and nurses passing by. We are waiting and looking for a bed on wheels to show up in the hallway. One of Dad's doctors comes into the room to inform us of the timing for Dad to be moved in an ambulance a couple of blocks away to Hospice.

"They should be here in about an hour." He leaves bowing with a smile, satisfied that he has fulfilled his task. Then we see Dr. Shah coming in to release Dad, as she said she would yesterday. Now, she walks over to my father's bed and puts her hand on his shoulder. She tells us that tests revealed that Dad has pneumonia.

She has a strong concern for his health. She suggests keeping him on an antibiotic for a few days until he gets better. And since Hospice can have no intravenous feeding, she wants to keep Dad right here where he is, in the cardiac unit until the pneumonia goes away.

That feels like another hard decision to make. Were we making the right decision?

I look over at Dad. He still seems ready to begin Hospice. My gut feeling is, *He'll heal once he's in Hospice.*

Honestly, Dad does not seem that sick to me. Somehow it does not seem like sticking around the cardiac floor is going to help. I feel strongly that this is the day for Dad to be transferred to Hospice.

They have a bed available. It is a small ward. There are no guarantees a bed will be there in a few days. Plus, I received the 'GO' code from the Lord.

My mother is sticking by her decision as well. We both feel led by the Holy Spirit to trust God and let them take Dad to Hospice that same day, as planned.

We tell Dr. Shaw how we feel. She reflects and comes up with her own answer, using her own logic.

"Yes, you are probably right. Without him being able to eat food, how effective would antibiotics be anyway?" she says. So she decides to make a counter offer.

She can help stop the inflammation in Dad's lungs by giving him a steroid shot into his IV. She takes the time to carefully do this and then leaves us with her blessing.

We, in turn, are grateful and feel good that we are sticking with our plan.

This whole time, Dad's nurse, Linda, is overseeing everything. She is standing inside the room by the doorway. The room becomes quiet again, and as we are waiting, there is stillness. To use a cliché, it is *pregnant*.

I am feeling like something more needs to happen. It seems to be an effort to break the silence. I feel the Lord urging me to speak.

"Talk to Linda, say anything!" comes a persistent inner voice.

I say the first thing I can think of, and ask her a simple question about her name. When I lived in France, I met many Africans, some spoke French while some spoke English. What about her? So I make the effort, and blurt out: "Are you from a country that speaks English. Is that why your name is Linda?"

Linda is relaxed and answers me. She tells us about her Nigerian background and that Linda is the name she uses as her English *middle name*. Her real first name (phonetically) is Ehe-Dena-Chi, which literally means "God has everything in his care."

All of a sudden, after breaking the commanding silence, we hear the joyful proclamation of our nurse telling us "God has everything in his care!"

For my part, I am nudging the Lord saying: "Thanks Lord! Wow, thanks. I'm glad I spoke up!"

Hearing our welcoming reception to her words, Ehe Dena Chi further explains that the names of each of her three brothers and three sisters all have the word "Chi" in them, which is the word for *God*.

"Kelli-Chi, is the name of my younger brother. 'Give thanks to God,' is what it means. My name means 'Everything is in God's care,'" she tells us again.

So, we forget we are waiting. I don't even notice or care about what is going on in the hallway. It feels more like we are being welcomed to join a celebration with our nurse, a humble Nigerian believer who seems deeply serious on the outside, but overflows from a well of joy, once a person with faith knows how to draw from it.

I think how affected by Ehe-Dena-Chi we all are. So different than what I am used to, as if she is God's gatekeeper for Dad. I'm so glad I spoke up because it is like being in a field that just looks like grass and then all these beautiful flowers blossom all around you, almost all at once. We are now in God's garden, about to go down a new beautiful path lined with flowers.

I think of Cillery, and the path there, lined with the most beautiful bushes and trees leading to a small paradise of fruitfulness, peaches, and strawberries. Yet, we're very much in the present moment, still very aware of the physical reality of the bed frame that my father is lying on and the tile floor I am standing on, aware that we are about to undertake my dad's final journey.

Whatever dread is in our hearts that could have been building up in the silence of the room, has been joyfully replaced by the proclamation of Dad's nurse Linda. By her very being, by her native name, Ehe-Dena-Chi is here to tell us, "Everything is in God's care."

Although this is a very difficult moment, especially for my mom, it is a moment when we all are changed and which clearly seems to have affected my father as well as we are drawn closer to the presence of Love.

Jesus said: "I will come to you. I will not leave you orphans." (John 14: 18 NKJ) We experience the inner strengthening of God's mighty Spirit which always produces joy. Even as we begin the journey of travelling with Dad on what will be his last days with us, we are surprised to find ourselves here, for an eternal moment, on this sunlit path surrounded by beautiful flowers. Yes, we are taking a step of no return, but this next step comes with more confidence, as Love has arrived to hold us up. What lies ahead will be better than I have imagined.

The hour goes by quickly. The outside hallway seems more friendly and secure because we are feeling more secure, after talking with Linda. And then, sure enough, like the next step in a dance, two transport girls come strolling through the door and take charge of the situation, graciously but firmly. One of the girls peels off Dad's oxygen sensor that is attached to his head; the second very lovingly takes out his IV needle. They carefully move Dad, with the help of a third nurse, and get ready to take him over to Hospice.

"Looks like there's going to be a big storm out there! Hospice is very close by. We sure want to get there before it starts pouring. But be assured, we will do our best to keep him dry," one of them tells us.

Just as they are leaving, the weather changes and becomes very turbulent outside the third-floor window. The wind starts howling and a big storm is breaking out. We can feel it everywhere.

The transport girls take off with Dad and we linger somehow, talking with Linda, thanking her, letting go and wrapping things up. Of course, we feel the awesomeness of the decision we have just made to take Dad off the IV, take Dad off all food and water, especially water.

When we get to Vitas, it is pouring rain. It is such a downpour that the only place we can see to park the car is the parking lot of the maternal fetus center next door. So here we are at the point of death, sitting out the downpour, looking at a sign that says *Maternal Fetus Center* and thinking about Life. About a little fetus not even born. Very humbling and very amazing.

HOSPICE

While we wait, we don't know what to expect. We are definitely a little apprehensive as we are about to enter this last leg of the journey.

The rain comes to a standstill and I re-park the car. We unlatch the iron gate and go up the short walkway and then down to the right under a big wide, long green awning. We come to a big wide door.

We need to press the buzzer to be admitted. I press the button.

"Come in," says a cheery voice as if we are expected for dinner. We enter into a wide long hallway that immediately differs from the hospital. The floors are made of real wood or laminate wood. They look soft, matte, not all shiny, and we barely have the time to take in more details because we are immediately greeted with a happy surprise. To the left of the entrance in this wide hall, the two kind transport girls are standing there with the now empty stretcher.

After traversing a deluge of rain, and waiting out the downpour in the Maternal Fetus parking lot, to see the two girls again is like a reunion of friends, and the best welcome we could have asked for.

"Hi!" we exclaim. "You're here! How did you make out?"

"Well, I'll tell you. We just made it before the downpour! We covered him up to protect him, and coming in he only had a couple of drops on his face; and as we entered here, he laughed!"

"He laughed!? Wow, that's great!" we say.

"Yes, he laughed. Even with the storm and the rain, and the few drops on his face. Once he was in here, he laughed."

"That's a good sign! Thanks for telling us."

"Yes, he is just down the hall to the right. They will show you to his room. We're off now, so all the best to you and your husband, Mrs. Swift."

"Thank you so much," responds my mother.

I haven't heard Dad laugh for over a week. What a good beginning to Dad's Hospice stay. I can hear that laugh and I take it as a sign of success. The manifestation of the joy in Dad can only be the confirmation that we connected with God's timing. How great to hear that laughter.

Dad's joy heralds more good news. Somehow, the pneumonia that made headway in him as he lay in the hospital bed did not come with him on this trip.

Right away we notice that his lungs are at peace. He is not coughing, not even a little bit. He is taking deep breaths. The pneumonia is gone.

Of course, our reaction is, "God healed Dad! He's not even coughing! We followed God's lead to bring him here and God took away the pneumonia in the process. See, everything worked out! We just had to follow the lead of the Holy Spirit! Wow, that's great."

Dad's room is set up for two people with a curtain drawn across the center. Dad is lying on his bed, which looks very much like a hospital bed, and he is resting peacefully. The other man is snoring slightly, though we cannot see him.

We meet the nurses, who are all very sweet and welcoming. The director comes in to welcome us and assures us they will be making sure that my father's stay is comfortable.

"His comfort is a high priority to us and we will be present and watching him around the clock."

The director introduces us to George, the nurse on night shift that evening. His winsome smile and confident demeanor present the very essence of the comfort the director has been talking about.

George makes a great first impression on me, and I immediately take a liking to him. He embodies a loving hug of caring with his great openness.

He naturally understands my urgent need to get water in my dad's mouth. He soon offers me a bag of foam pieces on sticks, used to clear out mucus gathering around the gums, or anywhere in the mouth.

George shows me how to clean out his mouth from built-up mucus using the sponge stick. He says he will help me with whatever I need.

In the drawer of my dad's room in Vitas Hospice for all of the days we are there, I can always be sure to find a steady supply of plastic bags filled with sponge sticks.

After cleaning out his mouth, I dip a fresh sponge stick into a small bottle of San Pellegrino and soak the water into the sponge. I gently put it against the inside of his cheek, or in the middle of his tongue. He sucks on the sponge, and to my amazement sometimes swallows small amounts, which makes me feel great that he is able to have water to drink. "Thank you, Jesus!" I exclaim.

Afterward, my father moves his head toward me in recognition for the relief the water brings him, and he looks at me with feelings of affection to thank me for keeping him hydrated.

The next afternoon my brother Greg comes to see Dad. He arrives at Hospice early that afternoon. Coincidentally, Fr. Walsh from St. Margaret Mary, my parent's church, also shows up. We are all standing around Dad. Fr. Walsh says affirming words and blesses him.

My Journal Entry:

Dad is lying very comfortably on his favorite left side. His head is down and sideways on the pillow. He looks tucked in, content, peaceful, sleeping at ease. Almost at home.

Greg walks in just as Nancy, the nurse, is done feeding Dad ice cream at my request and in my hopes that maybe he will swallow some. Greg arrives right before Fr. Walsh comes to visit.

After Fr. Walsh leaves us with some good cheer, Greg spends a long time contemplating Dad at his bedside. He puts his hand on his head and bends down to be near him.

Greg brought a card with a sailboat on it and he puts it on the night table for Dad.

I am standing at the foot of the bed watching and praying when Janice, my friend from Tulsa, calls me. I duck out, leaving Greg with Dad. So far Greg hasn't said anything to Dad and I hope this will be a special time for them, as Greg is leaving to go back to California in two days. It is great talking with Janice at this hour, so close to my Father's passing.

Come dinner time, we cross the street to the now familiar Outback restaurant. Greg and I share stories of living in Paris. Greg recalls with fondness our visits to Etretat, in Normandy, and the restaurant we always stopped at on the way there.

Mom is happy to connect with Greg again in person after seeing him last for Thanksgiving of 2012. Greg is staying at the Hyatt by the airport and spends all of Saturday with us. He says his final goodbye to Dad in Hospice on Sunday afternoon. I pray and hope he can have even a small connection with his father, as this will be his last time seeing him — and that he will be able to leave him feeling a sense of closure and of Dad's love.

I stay loyal to my mission to keep giving Dad water, holding a water-filled sponge stick in his mouth each time we are there, hoping the skin of his cheek or his tongue will absorb some water and he can maybe even swallow, and stay hydrated.

THANKS DAD

Tuesday. A lot happens during this day. Some quiet meditation holding Dad's feet, asking Jesus to show me the highlights of what my dad gave me. Maybe it is because of my empty stomach or God's presence during this sacred time, but Jesus shows me all right and makes me love my dad more.

What Dad taught me was all about all the cool things I could do with my body, like skiing and swimming. My dad taught me how to body surf, how to jump from one rock to another, how to land, how to climb, how to rappel, how I can be confident in the ocean, to find my balance in the waves, in the undertow, how to play in the sand, how to see God in the big spaces of the ocean, the starry expanse of the night sky, natural parks, the beauty of nature, how to run, run fast, the rhythm of Flamenco guitars and dancing, the love of animals, how to snorkel underwater, to enjoy the coral reefs, the beautiful colors of the fish and diving down to the ocean bottom and how to slowly release pressure on the way back up to the surface. Even to stand at the stern of the boat as it is cutting through the ocean waves, leaning over to the side, as the wind stretches the taut sails, how to ride a bike downhill knowing there might be cars coming at the cross-section and how I can still go fast, how to take risks and dive off the deck of my uncle Guy's sailboat in Corsica.

"Fearless," everyone said. "Marc is scared of nothing."

Thanks Dad.

ANGELS AT THE FINISH LINE

I just was a part of one of the most extraordinary life changing events of my life. Today is Mom's birthday, June 3. Mom and I are spending the afternoon celebrating with Dad. She has been able to let him go. Up until now, she hasn't wanted him to leave her. Mom had a very special quiet time with him yesterday and I feel that I have said everything to him that I have in my heart. Yesterday, she saw him struggling to breathe, making faces and having difficulty.

Today Mom tells me: "It is so hard for me to see Dad struggling to breathe. Each breath is such an effort for him! I just released Dad into Jesus' hands. I can let him go to Jesus now. I am happy for him that he can go home."

I think Dad knows she has let him go. Mom feels at peace.

This is the eleventh day of his long-distance marathon to the finish line. During this time, he cannot eat food, although fortunately, he can absorb a little water. The feelings he is used to having on long distance runs seem to be present, and he has stayed in good spirits. Dad is a real champion.

I feel a spirit of praise rising up within me and start singing "Therefore the Redeemed of the Lord," Dad's favorite gospel song. Mom is facing me on the other side of the bed and joins in. Dad is getting kind of a stereo effect as we sing on both sides of him.

"Therefore the redeemed of the Lord shall return,
"And come with singing,

"Unto Zion,
"And everlasting joy
"Shall be upon their heads.
"They shall obtain
"Gladness and joy!
"And sorrow, and mourning, shall flee away!
"Therefore the redeemed of the Lord shall return..."

What a perfect time to sing his favorite song — as he is about to receive everlasting joy upon his head! The singing feels right and one song becomes two and our singing leads into a bunch of songs, and we are singing songs he loves and songs that my mom loves. I am inspired and remember many songs of praise which I start up and my mom joins in, singing each song with joy and a smile.

We saturate the air around Dad and he seems happy and very relaxed. After at least a half hour of singing, I feel a sense of completion and we thank the Lord and say "Amen."

My mother excuses herself and leaves for fifteen minutes. I have a chair pulled up next to Dad on his right hand side, and this seems like a very special time. I sense a closeness to him. I pull out my cell phone and get ready to play him a Stevie Wonder song that is in my heart. I want him to feel the greatness of God's love.

"Dad, you know I love you, and God has always loved you. You are about to be with Him and enjoy His love for all eternity. Here is a beautiful song of God's love for you."

As around the sun the earth knows she's revolving,
And the rosebuds know how to bloom in early May
Just as hate knows love's the cure,
You can rest your mind assure,
That I'll be loving you always.
Always...

"Always" by Stevie Wonder

The song ends and the room is vibrant with a tangible presence of Life around us and between us. I say, "Dad, you are going to go to heaven soon and be with God who has always, always loved you and wants you to be with Him forever."

He looks at me with tenderness and I say: "I am proud of you, Dad. It's all good, Dad."

My mom comes back and puts her hand on my shoulder.

"I think it is time for us to leave."

I know that my father will go to heaven this evening, so it is hard for me to leave. I feel that this is all about my mom, and their marriage, and it is her husband. She does not want to see him die. Even though at many previous dinner times she told me she was grateful to be at the bedside of both her father and mother when they died.

We need to be in agreement, so I hug Dad and look at him close up and he gives me a smile and a nod.

It is a 'Go on, it's OK' look.

"See you later, Dad!" I say like I am not going far.

This exchange fits right in with my philosophy, so I am OK. Act like you are always with them and that you are coming back. Never say 'Goodbye' is my philosophy. It is too hard on the heart. Always say 'See you soon!' or 'I'll be back!' to a child or a grown-up or to a pet when you might be leaving for a while. So your presence stays peacefully with them.

Dad and I part with a hopeful heart.

Leaving is like a surreal experience for me, walking down the hall, out of the building, past the gate to the car parked on the curb. I feel like I am walking on air and am supported on both sides by a light-filled life force. The ride home is the same, I don't remember saying much. We left Dad in Donna's care and she says she will call us if Dad passes that night.

We are barely back in the apartment when we get her call. I am in the living room and Mom is in the kitchen when Donna calls. Mom tells me very slowly: "Dad just passed."

Is it a surprise? We feel upheld by a sense of love and light there with us. In God's grace, it all fits together; we are still dressed; it is 9:55pm, and the drive at night back to Hospice gives us time to absorb the news.

I drive back up Aloma to Lakemont with my mom. She said Donna told her an angel came to get my dad. There seems to be a lot of light around us — even though it is ten at night. I feel a great sense of peace.

We had just been there with Dad. Donna's story about an angel coming to get him captures our minds and hearts, and there is a sense of anticipation as we make our way back to the Vitas Hospice unit we left just twenty minutes ago.

We walk up to the door of Dad's room. Donna is there.

"Dad is laid out so well, so nicely," my mother says.

My dad's body is lying on the bed, all straightened out, under a clean covered blanket and sheet.

He's gone to heaven.

Donna tells us that she was there. She was there in the room when he passed. She saw him breathe his last breath. She said his eyes were staring intensely off into the distance, as if he was looking at something coming toward him over her right shoulder.

His gaze was so intense that she said, "What are you looking at?" to him, and even turned around to see who was there. She said his breathing was very serene; he was not laboring at all like he had been for the past two days.

Soon after he breathed his last breath, she felt the presence of angels in the room and such great peace and calm. It was wonderful.

My mom says to Donna: "I don't think the Lord wanted me to be here for his passing. It might've been too hard to see that."

Donna says, "Yes, and you know what, that is how it is so many times. The wife leaves, the family leaves, and he feels like it is OK to let go and go home now."

And that is what Dad did. He let go because he knew we were going to be OK, and he went home.

We thank Donna for how beautifully Dad is laid out and she says:

"Thank Winston because he's the one who really laid him out like that."

So we thank Winston and he says: "It all went smoothly."

Winston makes it sound like he oversaw my dad's journey to heaven — from the departure side *and* the arrival side!

'It all went smoothly?' I think, like Winston is an 'inside man.' An airline steward or a control tower operator, making sure the flights leave safely *and* arrive safely. Like Winston is saying: "He got there safely."

I think, *'Does God have special people to assist him with these very, very important transitions to eternity?'* I know that he must — now that I am face to face with Winston, a man who can see these transitions from heaven's viewpoint.

Winston can oversee the journey from earth to heaven, and he oversaw it for my dad. Wow! Thank you, Winston.

I am amazed. Looking up at the light shining on the ceiling between the two curtains next to us, I just keep thanking God and praising God's Glorious name for the peace everywhere, and it is so wonderful! Dad actually made it made it to heaven! It happened. It is such a good experience. While we are taking the time to appreciate our initial meeting with Donna and Winston, I feel a boundless joy, here in this place. Angels have been here! And they have left the feel of eternity here in the room.

I am so excited, I start jumping up and down three times.

I want to make a movie about it. I want to tell everybody: "It all works out! It is okay, if you know God, you can go there!"

I want to tell the whole world; it is such a wonderful experience. Angels have been in the room. Their presence is full of life and joy.

Donna later told me: "I've never seen anybody jump up and down like that! Your dad has just passed and you are jumping up and down because of all the joy in the room. I could feel it too; it was from the presence of the angels who had been there. Such life and joy. You had such a joyous smile knowing your father was at that moment looking into the face of Jesus. Your beautiful, elegant mother also felt the peace there. It has been a privilege to be a witness to your father's journey to heaven."

My mom says: "Isn't that wonderful, Marc, the way Dad went to heaven! You know what really touches me. I really have the feeling he waited before leaving so he could be here for my birthday."

"Yes Mom, he wanted to share your birthday with you!"

"Isn't that great?!"

LIFE AFTER DAD

My mom and I are very comforted in knowing that my father went to heaven so victoriously, with an angel coming to get him. We talk happily about our memories of Dad.

After Dad's death, there are a number of trials and tribulations regarding financial surprises and challenges, through no fault of my father's. I pray for a miracle right in keeping with all the extraordinary events we experienced with Dad.

The Lord turns everything around and Mom is back on her feet praising God. Even as we bounce back, I am aware of the very real grief that my mother now has to face. I believe it is very important for Mom not to be alone. Ever since my beloved son Josh died, I am very aware of how difficult it is to have a loved one leave even though they go to heaven.

My mom has much to plan with the details of the funeral arrangements, which is set a month after my dad dies. It is a joy to welcome the family from France when they come for Dad's memorial service. I take lots of pictures of this celebrative event. Everybody loved Uncle Bob, so there are many happy smiles from my dear cousins, Anne, Yann, Elise, and Simone. My father's brother Jonathan is there and his sister, Sandy. Jennifer and Elise are there with Greg and Heather. My mother sets out to make photographic packets to send to the family after they leave. It is great to see everyone.

In the pictures, I am aghast at how overweight I have become. Taking care of Dad and no longer being active detailing cars has taken a huge toll on me.

I start swimming in the Cloister's pool every day and my dedication pays off. I lose the weight after four months.

I live in the apartment with my mom for another six months. My mom asks me to keep writing the compilation of all her stories about her beloved father, 'Peré,' as she calls him. I have recorded our conversations on my phone, and add new ones which I later transcribe to my laptop. The book grows to include amazing war stories about her father in Lyon, their life in Cillery, her travels as a child on a boat liner between France and the USA, her father's textile business, her young adult years in Paris, and stories about meeting Bob and how much her parents liked him.

My mother is strong-willed and though I am here to help, she wants to do many things her way, or at least the same way she did them when she was on her own with Bob. Regardless of my dedication to my dad, my mother insists on making decisions independently of me. When her doctor is concerned about her lungs, she refuses to have diagnostic tests to determine ways to improve her health. Her doctor talks to her about the consequences of not acting soon. Though my mom can be stubborn, I stay present to accompany her on her journey.

Meanwhile, my friend, Janice, helps sell my house by making many interior design improvements. I trade my bright red Toyota Solara V6 convertible in exchange for her months of intensive work. As she works, she texts me pictures of the new kitchen, and new bathrooms. There is also a new generic carpet, to replace my original carpeting. For some reason the realtor did not think keeping my jaguar skin carpet would help sell the house.

By August, I receive a pod from Janice at my parent's storage place in Longwood with many of my belongings carefully packed.

My mom reluctantly relinquishes her twin beds by donating them to a local Catholic charity. For posterity, she passes on the oral history of the beds to the driver of the truck sent to pick up the items. She entrusts the historic beds into his care and waves goodbye to him when he leaves.

My new French friend, Fabrice, helps me rent a moving truck and we move Josh's bed, his computer desk and chair into my 'room.' The rest of my stuff, including the heavy jaguar carpet, are put into my newly rented storage unit.

I spend time with Fabrice, his wife and daughter and pray for the healing of many things in his life. He becomes a new creation in Christ Jesus, along with his wife and daughter. He wants to be baptized in the Church. The Lord opens the way for a priest from All Saints to baptize him and he renews his wedding vows.

Within six months following my father's death I meet Charlotte, a lady who goes to the Healing Service at All Saints Episcopal Church on Tuesday evenings. We have a great time and discover we have the same sense of humor and share the same values. By New Year's, I propose to Charlotte.

By January my mom wants her own space back and the Lord leads me to find an attractive apartment, within an eight-minute drive of my mother's location. My mom is happy for me and invites Charlotte and I to spend many Saturdays, sharing lunch with her and watching movies in the afternoons together. Sometimes we stay for a carry out dinner and a second movie.

I furnish the new apartment with the money from the sale of my house in Tulsa, and set up an audio booth to start work on narrating, recording and editing the audiobook of *The Coolness of Josh*.

Remember my friend Shon? My BMW X5 is still in Tulsa under Janice's care. I ask Shon if he would like to drive it to Florida for me and fly back to Tulsa. He loves the idea.

The day he arrives with my car, on January 19, 2014, Charlotte and I are there to greet him. He is so happy to see me again and to meet Char.

We spend a day at Disney World and have the greatest adventure together. My mom invites him to stay with her and he sleeps on Josh's bed, which my mom asked me to leave with her in the guest room, so the room is not empty. Their time together is invaluable as Shon and my mom share many faith stories. Shon thanks my mom for "their time of fellowship."

Two weeks later, Janice calls me to say that Shon has died of a heart attack. This begins a time of mourning for me, and Charlotte and I travel to Tulsa for Shon's Life Celebration service.

In 2010, I had to let go of my son, Josh, then six months ago my father and now my friend Shon? All Shon's friends are mourning and we have a warm reunion dinner with Mary, Janice, and more friends from Tulsa. Fortunately, Shon finished his life with a really happy time in Disney World before he went to heaven. I have a beautiful picture of Shon standing in front of the Magic Castle to put on the cards for the service and up on the screen in the church for everyone to see.

My mom is very encouraging and kind during the time after Shon's death. Her strong faith is always her greatest quality. There are seasons of joy between us but also difficult months of dementia when she feels very weak and wants to be by herself. I have a wealth of pictures and hours and hours of recordings on my cell phone of all our talks together.

Mom and I are very happy with our memories of Dad's new-found enthusiasm for living. She lives two and a half years after his passing before going to join him in heaven.

Thus ends the story of my father's escape from the isolation of Alzheimer's.

EPILOGUE

February 7, 2016. I just received a call from my Aunt Helen calling me from the beautiful nursing home in Switzerland where she lives. She calls to give me her condolences after the death of my mother. She and my mother were very close for a great number of years. Her call comes as a total surprise and I'm still taking in how great it feels.

Aunt Helen is the last living relative of my mother's generation. Although she has had a stroke, she is very positive and "Wonderful!" is her very uplifting, heartfelt response when she hears my voice on the phone. She already misses my mom.

She tells me: "Your mother was a wonderful woman."

"Yes, Aunt Helen, she was a wonderful woman," I say. "She is very happy to be back with Bob now."

Yes, this marks the end of an era. Aunt Helen stands tall as the last representative of her generation. My mom died January 8, 2016. She died peacefully, after a sudden onset of pneumonia, and being put on a respirator. As she lay in the hospital bed, she had the face of a lion or of an eagle, a young looking face that reflected the great strength that she held in an increasingly weakened body.

Now my mom is reunited with her bear, "mon ours."

I am glad kid Marc is still with me to share the story.

"I love how Dad escaped the prison of the Alzheimer's and reconnected with us. How are we going to end this story?" says kid Marc.

I take my orator's pose and brandish my arm, saying, "Thus a story that could have ended badly...ends well! All's well that ends well."

"The story did end well. An angel coming to get him. That is a happy ending," says kid Marc laughing and smiling at me.

"That is a happy ending!" I say.

"We reached his heart," says kid Marc.

"And Dad reached back with love," I reply. "Thank you, Jesus."

I knew what kid Marc was going to say next, so as soon as he starts to say it, I join in and we say it together: "Reach the love in the heart and the heart will reach back with love!"

"Well done, kid Marc!" I say.

"That's the heart of the matter, in the end," says kid Marc.

"Are you trying to be funny?"

"I'm putting my finger on the pulse, that's all."

"You're beating me when it comes to the humor," I quip back.

"I'm taking this to heart!"

"Reach out and touch the heart, right?" I say. "We reached out to Dad and he reached back!"

"With the love," says kid Marc.

"With the love, that's right! What happened to the dictator? Where did he go?"

"He got left behind. Too heavy for the ride."

"Like the airlines. Way over 50 pounds. Too heavy and no fun," I say.

"Deadly," kid Marc adds.

"We outwitted him," I say.

"With God's help," says kid Marc. "If God is for us, who can be against us?!"

"Yes, love conquers all," I say. "Love will find a way."

"We found the way!" exclaims kid Marc. "We reached his heart!"

"And Dad reached back with love!" I say, hugging kid Marc.

THE END

ABOUT THE AUTHOR

M ARC SWIFT, author, speaker, father, is no stranger to pain. Marc writes and speaks of his miraculous healing of a brain tumor after being given only five years to live. Since this healing, his passion for helping others with restoration through Jesus has continued and grown.

Rescuing his son, Josh, from near suicide and restoring him to a happy life and the love of God his Father was Marc's greatest accomplishment. After his son's peaceful death in 2010, he wrote his first book, The Coolness of Josh and the subsequent color workbook, New Joy and Peace after Childhood Abuse. Marc's creative talent in writing and voice presentation is showcased in the dynamic audiobook version of his book.

Marc was a successful small business entrepreneur running an auto detail company with his sons in Tulsa, Oklahoma, for 25 years. In 2012, he moved to Winter Park, Florida, to help his mother care for his father who had Alzheimer's Disease. From Alzheimer's With Love is the result of this remarkable journey in the pursuit of healing his father through the grace of Jesus.

He studied Art, French, and Literature in England and Film at Brown University graduating in 1980. Raised in Paris, France, and England until the age of 20, Marc currently resides in Oviedo, Florida, and is engaged.

CPSIA information can be obtained
at www.ICGtesting.com
Printed in the USA
FFOW04n0118100317
33211FF

9 781613 398784